	CLACTON	- JAN 2018
- 3 FEB 2018		
13 FEB 18		
1 5 MAR 2018		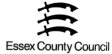 D0589941

Please return this book on or before the date shown above. To renew go to www.essex.gov.uk/libraries, ring 0345 603 7628 or go to any Essex library.

Essex County Council

RE-NOURISH

RHIANNON LAMBERT

Harley Street Nutritionist

A Simple Way to Eat Well

yellow
kite

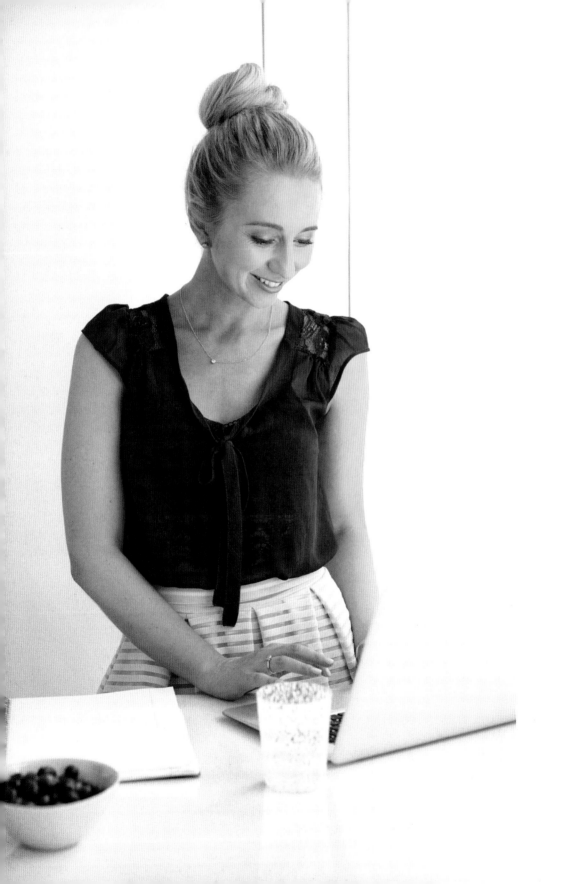

CONTENTS

BIOGRAPHY

Rhiannon Lambert is a nutritionist specialising in weight management, eating disorders and sports nutrition. She is the founder of Rhitrition, a leading Harley Street private clinic.

As a professional soprano who trained at the Royal Academy of Music (she won Classic FM's Young Musician of the Year at the age of 17), Rhiannon learned early on the importance of living a healthy lifestyle. Her belief that nutrition can play a significant role in your overall health, wellbeing and appearance has been tested as she has performed all over the world.

Registered with the Association for Nutrition (AFN), Rhiannon obtained a first-class Bachelor (BSc) degree in Nutrition and Health and a Master's (MSc) degree in Obesity, Risks and Prevention. She also has diplomas in Nutritional Interventions, and Excellence in Practitioner Skills for Eating Disorders. Her qualified approach to nutrition and total dedication to her clients' needs has seen Rhiannon work with some of the world's most influential people.

Creative in her approach to ingredients, she has won over *Masterchef's* Gregg Wallace and is responsible for developing menus at London's most celebrated healthy eateries, such as The Detox Kitchen. Rhiannon has also worked with Olympic athletes, witnessing the dramatic impact nutrition can have on performance at the highest level and showing that food and fitness should work together to keep us in peak condition. Additionally, her experience working alongside cardiologists and general practitioners at NHS hospitals has seen her demonstrate the influence nutrition has in metabolic syndrome and recovery.

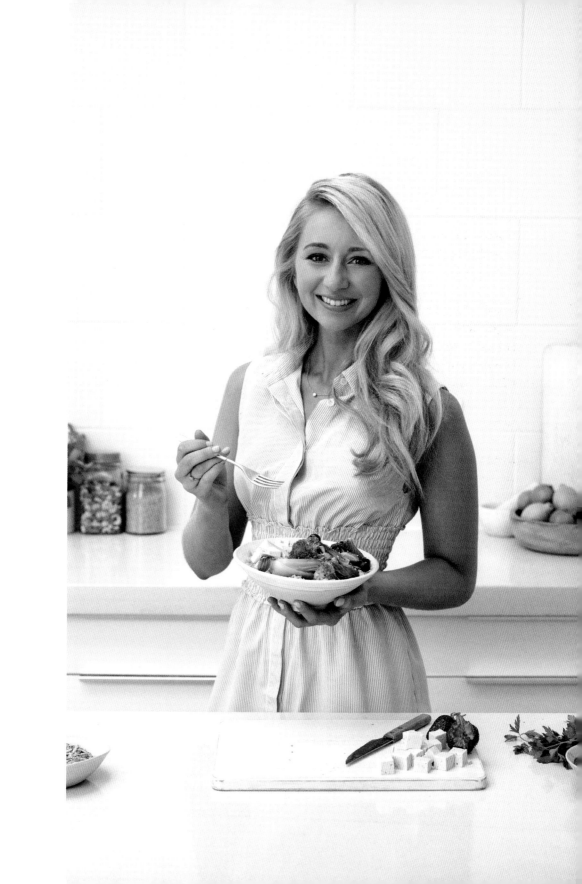

MY STORY

I grew up in an unassuming town in Wiltshire with little opportunity – only a love for musical theatre ensured I didn't fall in with the wrong crowd at school. I dreamed of performing on stage and the fact that I could sing gave me my only confidence.

As a teenager, I worked hard to pursue my musical ambitions, making foot-long sandwiches in Subway and working as a kitchen maid in the local all-girls boarding school, a place that seemed a world away from my reality. Evenings and weekends were filled with amateur dramatics – all while trying to maintain an academic record. Having won a national singing competition at 15, my friends encouraged me to audition for what had previously only been a fantasy: Classic FM's Young Musician of the Year. To my amazement, I won – aged just 17 and without any formal classical training.

Achieving well beyond any expectations, I immediately left home to sign with a major record label and embark upon on a whole new life in London. It was a daunting challenge and I began living a somewhat double life, where I performed at glitzy Mayfair locations and mingled with the rich and famous, yet walked home to a rundown London council estate.

Thrust into the limelight, I worked with Coldplay's vocal coach, sang on stage with Alfie Boe, was praised by Michael Ball and got standing ovations from Simon Cowell. I was singing in front of everyone from international royalty to Peter Andre, S Club 7 and Boyzone. I was really led to believe that I would be the next Katherine Jenkins. But it was not to be. After three years of relentless songwriting and singing, financed by odd jobs including stewarding at the Royal Albert Hall, I was told that the recession meant record labels were no longer willing to speculatively invest in new talent. Following a second unsuccessful stint with another record label, I was left with a singing career over before it had even started.

During my time in the music industry, the pressures of looking a certain way had persuaded me to follow restrictive and unsustainable diets. The record industry's pursuit of me achieving overnight changes by quick fixes held no boundaries. Believing that shop-bought diet products and meal replacement drinks were the answer to looking your best, I began to suffer from malnourishment; my energy levels were so low that I went to my GP for answers. Instead of identifying my nutritional deficiencies, he prescribed me anti-depressants which I naively began to take. I had never been confident about my appearance before but this was a particularly low point in my life. When I was performing, I regularly witnessed the destructive impact of disordered eating among other aspiring performers. I was given inadequate, unqualified advice and listened more and more to it as I held onto any hope left for my disappearing singing career. With all my friends already graduating from university and seemingly living life to the full, I felt left behind, trapped in a fantasy world where I had no control.

I started to take more of an interest in nutrition to reinvigorate me and my life and soon realised this was my true calling. As soon as I made the life-changing decision to enrol at university as a mature student to study nutrition, I knew just how important it was for me to unlearn everything I thought I knew. I endeavoured to learn from my mistakes and become as qualified as possible – no easy feat for someone coming at human science from a musical background! In fact, I felt like I had to work ten times harder than those who already had a scientific educational background.

After a gruelling three years, I proudly obtained a first-class degree in Nutrition and Health from the University of Roehampton; my insatiable interest in learning pushed me to immediately enrol in a Masters degree in Obesity, Risks and Prevention.

After a total of four years at university, funded by a stream of odd jobs worked at all hours of the day, I sought as much work experience as possible as I looked to embark upon a career in nutrition. Straight out of university, I was managing a café part-time for a boutique fitness studio, advising gym goers on optimal pre- and post-workout nutrition, as well as interning at a number of leading health brands including The Food Doctor. A few months later a chance meeting with a healthy food delivery company saw me working in their kitchen devising recipes for their A-list clients. Meanwhile, I was introducing myself to every practising nutritionist and clinic in town. My proactive approach soon paid off when I was given an unimaginable opportunity to work in a private health clinic in London's respected Harley Street.

Working alongside a full team of GPs, cardiologists and other medical professionals, I supported the clinicians who were working with private clients. Listening to the ways in which all these highly trained and experienced professionals were able to shape people's lives, I realised more than ever the importance of continuing my professional development. Having gone on to study further in eating disorders, I quickly found myself attracting a diverse clientele. In early 2016, with the rise in social media and a waiting list for private consultations, I founded my own Harley Street clinic called Rhitrition – a combination of Rhiannon and nutrition. I wanted to help people learn how to re-nourish their bodies.

Words cannot express how grateful I am to all those who have supported me in my career so far. Nothing is more important than what we eat, so I am absolutely delighted to have been given the opportunity the share my nutritional knowledge and expertise far beyond my Harley Street clinic in the form of this, my first book. I feel privileged to be a part of the growing wellness movement that demands qualified experts as the authoritative voices for our nutrition and health. With an evidence-based understanding of what nutrition really means to your mind and body, *Re-Nourish* will help build the foundations for a happy, healthy relationship with food and get you back to basics with a simple approach to eating well, for life.

TESTIMONIALS

'Can't recommend her enough, the best nutritionist in town. Thank you for leading us to a healthy lifestyle.'

CESC FABREGAS & DANIELLA SEAMAAN – PROFESSIONAL FOOTBALLER & MOTHER

'No fads, no gimmicks, just beautiful healthy food. Eating this way really helps you get the most from everyday life – a must for me and my family!'

CATHERINE TYLDESLEY – *CORONATION STREET* ACTRESS

'Rhiannon understands that it is about so much more than diet. It's not just about tidying up the outside, she looks at the whole person and really gets under the bonnet! There are no gimmicks. I couldn't recommend her highly enough.'

RONNIE O'SULLIVAN – OBE, PROFESSIONAL SNOOKER PLAYER

'I couldn't recommend Rhiannon more highly. She is so incredibly passionate about educating and equipping both men and women with the tools to build themselves a healthy and sustainable way of eating that is the complete antithesis of the diet culture we find ourselves surrounded by each day.'

ALICE LIVEING – BESTSELLING AUTHOR AND PERSONAL TRAINER

'I know Rhiannon professionally and personally. She is bright, charming and clever. I look forward very much to working with her again.'

GREGG WALLACE – *MASTERCHEF*

'Rhiannon has an amazing understanding of nutrition through years of study and makes it easy to follow. If you're going to invest in your health, I would recommend her as the perfect guide.'

DAVID SMITH MBE – PARALYMPIAN GOLD MEDALLIST ROWER

'Rhiannon has helped me completely overcome my digestive issues. She is so helpful and always goes that little bit further. It's so refreshing to work with someone who really understands your problems and can help you solve them.'

TIFFANY WATSON – *MADE IN CHELSEA* ACTRESS

'Having Rhiannon's support has been invaluable. She's helped me understand my exact nutritional needs as an athlete, how to increase energy levels and as a result has helped me perform at my very best.

WILL BAYLEY – PARALYMPIAN GOLD MEDALLIST TABLE TENNIS PLAYER

'One of the very few practitioners that I highly recommend. A high level of expertise combined with experience working in a very complex and emotive field make Rhiannon one of the UK's leading specialists, and the only one I would call on.'

DALE PINNOCK – THE MEDICINAL CHEF

'Rhiannon has shown me how to enhance my performance through nutrition and shop effectively. She is always there when I need advice.'

NICK COMPTON – ENGLAND INTERNATIONAL CRICKETER

'Working with Rhiannon gave me the information and inspiration to make smarter food choices and to listen better to the nutrition needs of my own body.'

JUSTIN SOMPER – BESTSELLING AUTHOR

'Rhiannon is a brilliant and effective nutritionist because she is incredibly knowledgable and yet also, incredibly relatable, making it easy to absorb her food and diet philosophy. She is science with a smile and I have learned so much from our time together.'

SHONA VERTUE – PERSONAL TRAINER AND AUTHOR
OF *THE VERTUE METHOD*

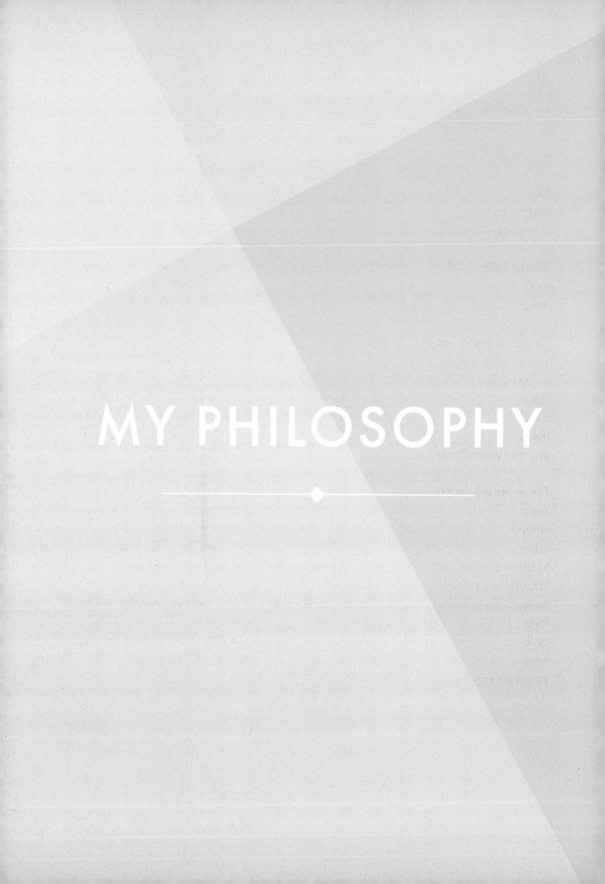

MY PHILOSOPHY

Our bodies really are as unique as our personalities, so each of us should strive to find a way of eating that works for us individually. I believe in empowering everyone to embrace a healthy way of living through the food we enjoy and the life we lead.

Almost half of all Brits have tried to lose weight at some point, with the figure rising to as high as 57 per cent for just women. And almost two-thirds of dieters say that they are pretty much on a diet 'all or most of the time'.[1]

Large numbers of you have experimented with dieting in some shape or form; some of you may have even made some more drastic changes to the way you eat. If you have, it is likely that you will have seen some results, at least in the short term. But what faddy diet peddlers don't share is that the true measure of a diet isn't how you feel hours, days or even weeks later; it's how you feel after months and years. There are a lot of non-evidence-based 'diets' or fads out there that try (and often succeed) to convince you that you will lose weight healthily when, in fact, the opposite is true.

The social media obsession with meals presented as art has turned food into fashion. I want to bring the focus back to nutrition, so that you can eat well and cook what you want. I am of the firm belief that getting back to basics and keeping nutrition simple is the easiest way to maintain a healthy lifestyle in the long term. I'm really excited to share my vision of food as something that should always be a positive aspect of life, offering enjoyment, fuel and happiness for both the mind and body. There are no quick fixes and what works for some may not work for others. No food should be forbidden and we need to stop thinking of certain foods as being intrinsically 'good' or 'bad.' I believe there is absolutely no place for restriction or the elimination of whole food groups in a healthy relationship with food. Instead of focussing on what you can't eat, focus on what you can and should be eating.

For anyone on the brink of trying another diet or giving up on one, let me assure you I have been there too: confused and lost, feeling trapped and unsure how to get out. The answer is easier than a lifetime of searching for something that doesn't exist. Anything is possible when you look at things from a different angle.

The key to good health isn't hiding in a fad diet and you definitely won't find it in any supposed superfood. The answer doesn't lie in subscribing to yet another diet or more rules to follow. I want you to live a life where food has no power over you, except to bring you nourishment and joy.

Remember: health isn't immediately repairable and weight isn't immediately modifiable. The idea that some new food discovery or new way of combining food will give you an instant fix to your weight or health problem is misinformed; there is no overnight fairy-tale ending. Weight loss at speed is never a good idea – slow and steady is the way to go.

Part of the journey to gaining a healthy relationship with food is to acknowledge that eating is a chance to nourish. It shouldn't be that you must eat this or that way, or only ever choose to eat certain foods. Each and every one of us is different with unique nutritional requirements. The foods that are best for you might not be best for your spouse, friend or child. Personal tastes, natural shapes and sizes, genetics and so much more influence what foods will and won't benefit us.

The idea of nourishing your mind and body works because it's not a diet or a quick fix: it's a way of life. Soon enough, the tips and tricks I've shared in this book, and which form the core of good nutritional eating, will become second nature to you, helping you to become the healthiest version of yourself. Having the knowledge and tools to put healthy eating into action are really the only things necessary to achieve your health goals. In the following chapters, I will reveal to you many of the methods and elements I use when working with clients in my clinic. Think of it as your back-to-basics guide, full of supportive resources from mindful eating techniques, a nutritious weekly menu, portion guidelines and answers to the most popular questions I get asked in my clinic.

Just as I did, I would like you to consider unlearning everything you thought you knew about nutrition. Try to start with a fresh outlook on exploring what will work best for you as an individual. With an enthusiastic mindset and a belief in the power of positive nutrition, I can show you the difference between feeling merely okay and feeling on top of the world. And whatever anyone tells you, optimum nutrition is ultimately about eating with pleasure and without shame.

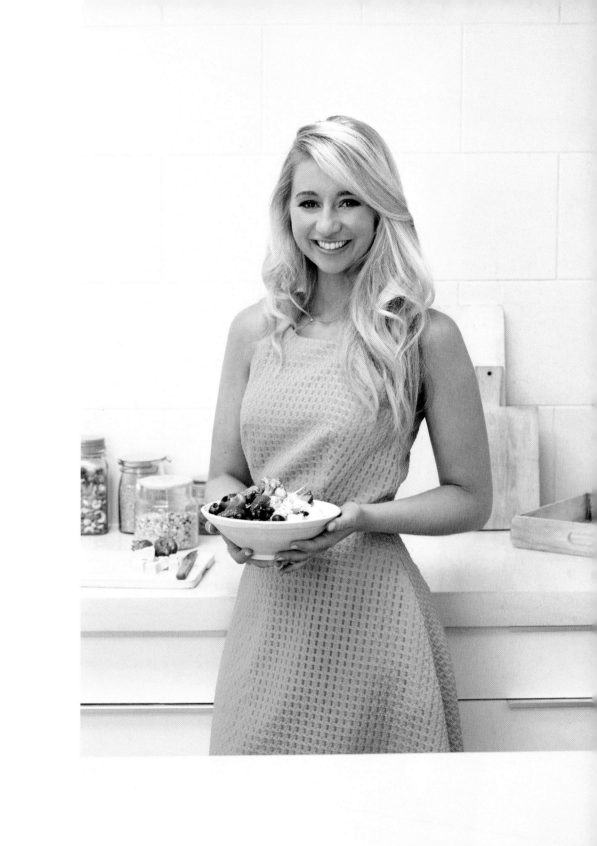

KNOWLEDGE NOT MAGIC

Every single client I see longs for me to wave a magic wand or prescribe a miracle pill. Quick fixes and short-term plans may sound exciting, creating hope and the idea of happiness in next to no time, but all they tend to do is give you just a glimpse of those dreams – until suddenly they don't. Faddy diets are notoriously hard to maintain; what is more, although you may see some immediate weight loss, their impact on your mind and body in the longer term is not known.

The unsustainable and (usually) unhealthy nature of quick fixes means that they often create a yo-yo effect too, leaving you frustrated. All too many people give up on healthy regimes, accepting that their struggle with food is just a part of how their life is and will always be.

But it really doesn't have to be this way.

Instead of wishing for overnight success, consider your path to healthy eating and an enriched mind and body as a journey, where a basic nutritional education is the key to taking that first step and staying on the right track. After all, if you don't know how or why you've got somewhere, how can you expect to stay there? Knowledge is power, as they say.

NUTRIENTS NOT NUMBERS

Being aware of the calorie content in food has long been drummed into us and those who try to lose weight often use a total daily calorie intake as a guide to what they can and can't eat. The thing is, calories really aren't much more than a number and we shouldn't be relying on calorie content to dictate what constitutes a healthy diet. Calories can be deceptive and very damaging when used inappropriately.

There is a bizarre concept that suggests that a calorie is a calorie; that its impact on our body is the same regardless of its form. In a world full of heavily processed foods, how on earth can a calorie in one food be the same as any other? It's common sense to understand that 100 calories of chocolate biscuits will most certainly not have the same impact as 100 calories of broccoli.

Calculating and planning every single meal and restricting what you really want to eat based on calorie counting is not going to nourish your mind and body. Furthermore, the trend of macro counting has only confounded any confusion about the effectiveness of calorie counting. If you're not familiar with macros (short for macronutrients), they represent the amount of protein, carbohydrates and fat in the foods we eat. Counting macros down to the very last gram forgets that we may not need exactly the same amount of macronutrients every single day of the year. Our bodies really are incredible things and our needs constantly change; by tracking macros we are unable to keep up with and honour these daily differences, not to mention the fact that we are ignoring all the essential micronutrients we need to thrive (see page 40 for more on these).

THE FOUR 'R'S

Regardless of any ailment or specific concerns, I ask every client of mine in clinic to see food as nourishment and something that affects both your mind and body. For me, nutrition, movement, mindset and rest are the four pillars of health. And with many of my clients leading active lifestyles, I ask them to follow four easy-to-remember principles:

R   Respect. You and your body deserve the best, so make it a priority to see eating as an opportunity to nourish. If you treat your body right, it will treat you right.

R   Refuel. Don't waste your time being active without properly refuelling your body with nutrition. You really can't train your way out of a bad diet.

R   Rehydrate. The human body is actually about 60 per cent water so it makes perfect sense that we need to keep our levels topped up. Too many of us are simply not drinking enough.

R   Recover. Recovery encompasses more than just muscle repair. Recovery involves restoring your chemical and hormonal balance, nervous system, mental state and so much more. Don't ignore your body when it needs to be rested.

LISTEN TO YOUR BODY

In my experience, too many people look to others to tell them what will work for their body instead of listening carefully to their own individual needs and instincts. This is such an important issue to address and one of the most underestimated and challenging tasks I set in my clinic. No one is smarter than your own body when it comes to knowing what you truly need. I teach my clients how to learn the skills to tune into your body's requirements, putting emotion and judgement to one side. Learning to listen to your body's cues so you address its fundamental needs – free from emotion or habit – will enable you to quickly form a much healthier relationship with food.

Your body is equipped to know when you have had enough food so there's no need to meticulously monitor every morsel that you put into it. It has built-in cues to tell you when to eat and when to stop eating. The practice of engaging all of our senses to guide our eating-related decisions is what I look to achieve with all of my clients. It really is empowering to eat intuitively.

A HEALTHY RELATIONSHIP WITH FOOD

Everyone has a unique and special relationship with food. It can be a powerful thing when used effectively for mind and body but, if abused, it can also be detrimental to our health. Food should never be a source of guilt and exercise should never be about counteracting what we ate earlier or punishing ourselves for eating. We all need food to sustain ourselves, and even if we indulge at times, it doesn't mean we should feel bad or see it as any kind of weakness – food is to be enjoyed! The key to taking any advice on healthy eating and nutrition is to remain open-minded. Being too rigid, restrictive or strict about nutritious eating can cause problems.

In an ever-demanding and increasingly stressful world, the mindfulness boom has never been more important. This is something I work on with every single one of my clients because it's at the very core of a healthy body. Ordinary life often means we feel stressed. Our minds whizz away tackling difficult, confusing emotions or work and family pressures, and at times it feels as if we don't really know how to deal with them. We are often so distracted by what's going on around us that we are no longer truly present in the world in which we live and we miss out on the things that are most important to us. But that's really not how it has to be!

Our nutrition deserves at least equal thought and consideration as the many chores we complete each day. I admit this is a challenge – I too have to stop myself from rushing my food while working at my desk, or when I've just walked through the door at the end of the day. I always remind my clients that the food we eat has to undergo a complex biological process in the body, which takes time and involves a lot more interactions than a simple mouth-to-stomach pathway. Even if you consume the healthiest of diets, if your digestion isn't working optimally, any nutrition won't be put to good use and sadly you won't see all the potential benefits. And good digestion starts with taking the time to eat properly and mindfully (see pages 82–6 for more on this).

Mindful eating can also help to combat and understand emotional eating. Every day I work with clients suffering from various forms of eating distress, so I know exactly how food is often intertwined with our emotions; sadness often makes us eat less but more commonly it causes us to overeat items that are high in fat and sugar, such as chocolate and cakes, which we all commonly view as comfort foods. But you do not need to label yourself as an emotional eater to emotionally eat. For some reason, we are conditioned to crave positive reinforcement when we do something well, and there's a huge temptation to reward ourselves with – often unhealthy – food. They say food is the most-used drug for anxiety but I want you to see food as a way to fuel your body properly so that you can feel good, look good, and live your life to the fullest.

Being more aware of whether or not you are falling into mindless eating traps, restrictive dieting cycles, bingeing, guilt and shame or any black-and-white thinking will enable you to proactively make changes to these thought processes. It won't happen overnight but learning to eat mindfully is one part of the puzzle that can be solved. I often work alongside a counsellor or psychologist with some of my clients as I find it enhances progress and recovery.

FIND YOUR HAPPY PLACE

There is now more pressure than ever before to be healthy and yet we seem to have lost the concept of balance and any happy in-between. We should all be encouraging and supporting each other to live a lifestyle that makes us feel great and feel comfortable with the food we eat every day.

Lead your life free from social comparisons, poor health, low mood and a terrible diet. Just because someone influential has decided to give up something or follow a trend doesn't make it the right move for you, just as if you are a vegan or a vegetarian no one should dictate how you should change your personal lifestyle choice. I want to empower you to make the right choices for only you and no one else. Do what you can and at your own pace. Comparison really is the thief of joy. So, let's embrace our individualities and re-nourish ourselves with a nutritional education.

STEP OFF THE SCALES

Start your journey by stepping off those scales, which I call The Sad Step. For me, it was honestly life-changing. It cannot be denied that weight does offer us some useful measure, but weighing yourself too often can cause anxiety, distress and can even dictate your mood for the day. At worst it can even cause a spiral of deprivation, binge eating and low self-esteem.

Instead try to focus on yourself and not obsess about any particular weight or number. So many of us pin our happiness and mark our success based on a number on the scales, but it should never be to the extent that our self-worth, value and significance rests on it. Anyone who has dieted will fully appreciate that achieving their perceived perfect weight rarely brings the happiness and feelings of self-fulfilment that they had hoped for. Being the 'right' weight unfortunately doesn't take life's problems away.

Before the arrival of body weight scales we managed to maintain our weight without knowing what it was. Now too many of us wake up every morning, jump on the scales and adjust our day according to the number we see. If you are that person, what does that tell you? Ask yourself, is it making you happy? Is it really enhancing your quality of life? Or is it sometimes holding you back from the events you then had planned that day?

The human body is one incredibly complex piece of machinery. There are things going in and coming out; it's transforming all the time. As a result, your weight can easily fluctuate over the course of a 48-hour period. Depending on what you ate, how much water you drank, whether you ate lots of salty foods and what time of day you weighed yourself, your weight is likely to be quite different.

If binning the scales is a step too far for you, just start by moving your weigh-ins to weekly, then fortnightly and then less often. Do what feels right for you but don't be a slave to the scales.

FIGHT THE FADS

Research by supermarket Sainsbury's found that more than a fifth (21 per cent) of young people refer to social media, YouTube stars and bloggers to find information on healthy eating; while 44 per cent of young people think that cutting out a whole food group can promote a healthy lifestyle.[2] This is concerning, since many of those social media stars are not qualified nutritional experts and, as such, their advice is not monitored, so can be misleading or simply wrong. You'll rarely find mention of a nutritional degree, which teaches the evidence-based biochemistry, physiology, pathophysiology and psychology required to be able to safely advise what someone should and shouldn't be eating.

Practising health professionals like me, by virtue of our relationship with our clients, have a duty of care. We are bound by a code of conduct and ethics approved by government legislation. I actually believe self-proclaimed health bloggers are doing nothing wrong by encouraging healthy eating, yet with their immeasurable influence, surely there has to be a responsibility to ground their promises in evidence. Above all else, no matter what qualifications or lack thereof, we should all be deeply suspicious of pseudoscience, when claims are presented as being plausible or 'scientific', but are not justifiable by science or fact.

Most of us would like to be healthier and learning about food should always be encouraged. Unfortunately, as long as the term 'nutritionist' remains legally unprotected, anyone can call themselves a nutritionist regardless of whether or not they have any formal training, while many doctors and GPs are frustrated that nutrition doesn't form part of their existing medical training. It's never been more important to approach the right health professionals and for us all to work together and collaborate in the best interests of the public.

STAY MOTIVATED

Every now and again, we all need some motivation to get us going. I hope this book will inspire you to live a healthier way of life but if you're still unsure, know that eating better will ensure you are at a much lower risk of needing to rely on doctors and medicine to maintain your health. Just some of the benefits include higher energy levels, lower cholesterol and blood pressure and reduced sickness.

However, the higher the expectations you set, the greater the risk of stopping any plan within the first 12 months. Having realistic expectations increases your chances of maintaining a healthy lifestyle. Also, if you put pressure on yourself to achieve any health goal too quickly, your overall health will suffer, so remember to take it one step at a time. There is the goal-setting theory called S M A R T, which can help us set better goals – you will probably have come across it at work but it is just as useful in all areas of life. It states that for a goal to be truly motivating, it should be:

Specific
Measurable
Attainable
Realistic
Timely

What this means is a clear and easily measureable goal that is realistic for you and set within a specific timeframe. Vague goals of 'losing weight' or 'eating more healthily' do not subscribe to the S M A R T goal rules, whereas 'I will eat 5 portions of vegetables every day' or 'I will work out 3 times a week' do. By creating goals that meet these criteria, you will significantly increase the success rate of achieving them and you may even get superior results.

Remembering exactly why you are making healthy choices will also help you stay on course. It really is helpful to make a list of specific reasons why you want to get healthier. Why not keep your list on your phone so you can check it whenever you need a quick boost to stay on track?

A FINAL NOTE

I'm always reminding my clients just how incredible our bodies are but one thing we simply cannot do is turn rubbish into a high-quality product. All of our cells, muscles, skin, bones – I mean everything – are built from the food that you supply it, so please choose wisely whenever you can.

As long as you believe in the power of positive nutrition and make informed choices to nourish your mind and body more often than not, you should live a long and fulfilling life with few health concerns.

If anything you read, hear or see is confusing, please consult a qualified health professional. A bit of extra guidance and advice may be all it takes to help you become the healthiest and happiest version of you.

I hope you too believe in my philosophy and approach to nutrition. I can assure you that everything I say and do is achievable and can have a positive effect on your mind and body. I am living proof of it and if this book has once single objective, it is to arm you with the basic knowledge to enable you to make educated and informed choices about the food you eat.

Good luck! Keep in touch with #ReNourish ⓘ 🐦 f @Rhitrition

NOURISHMENT

The word nourishment has been thrown around for so long that its true meaning has been somewhat lost.

Ultimately, nourishment means getting everything your body needs from your diet to perform optimally. It doesn't mean you have to lose weight or follow the latest diet fad to feel good about yourself.

The likes of eating clean, going gluten-free and giving up carbs may sound compelling in their promises for quick results, but these are simply nothing more than restrictive diets that may cause long-term damage as a result of limiting the range of nutrients your body receives. Trust me, I know and have been there.

In order to achieve optimum nutrition – which is crucial to a healthy state of mind – you need to return to the basic principles of evidence-based nutrition and learn what works for you as an individual. You are unique and will require something different to the person next to you.

Aim to consume natural, whole foods most of the time as these are often great sources of nutrients, whereas heavily processed foods usually offer less nutritional value. Processed foods aren't just microwave meals and other ready meals: the term 'processed food' applies to any food that has been altered from its natural state in some way. This means you may be eating more processed food than you realise. Processed foods aren't always unhealthy, but anything that's been processed may contain added salt, sugar and fat. One advantage of cooking food from scratch at home is that you know exactly what is going into your meals. Basing your diet on natural, whole foods is an extremely effective yet simple strategy to quickly improve and maintain good health.

UNDERSTANDING MACRONUTRIENTS

There are three macronutrients: carbohydrates, fat and protein. All of these are required in relatively large amounts each day and each support vital functions in your body. Quite simply, these three macronutrients give your body the energy it needs.

Even the most simple of tasks such as breathing requires energy so don't underestimate the power of good nutrition. Like me you may be sitting behind a desk all day, not physically moving, but your brain still requires fuel, which is why you'll often feel peckish when devoting a lot of thought to anything. You need to also take into account your daily activity – the more rigorous it is, the higher the energy expenditure and the more energy your body will require to keep working optimally. And please remember: there is no one-size-fits-all solution in nutrition. Your optimal intake of each macronutrient depends on numerous factors including age, gender, genetics, physical activity and personal preferences. All of these individual differences will affect the amount of energy you need to consume.

STOP SHAMING CARBOHYDRATES

Cutting carbohydrates was once hailed as the answer to fast track health and weight loss. The Atkins and so many other diets all avoid bread, potatoes and pasta in favour of loading up on protein sources and high-fat items. These popular diets only heightened the already widespread misconception that carbs make you gain weight. However, the view that all carbs should be cut from someone's diet is quite simply wrong.

Carbohydrates hold a special place in nutrition as they provide the largest single source of energy in the diet. Most carbs get broken down or transformed into glucose, which can be used as energy. Carbs can also be turned into fat (stored energy) for later use. Glucose is the essential fuel for our brains and the preferred energy source for our muscles during strenuous exercise. If you're naturally lean and physically active, a diet rich in carbohydrates is likely to enhance your performance and lifestyle.

GLYCEMIC INDEX (GI) AND GLYCEMIC LOAD (GL)

You may have come across these terms but not known exactly what they mean. Glycemic index (GI) is a measure that tells you how quickly a carbohydrate food will make your blood glucose levels rise after eating it. The higher the GI, the faster the impact. Low GI foods are more slowly digested, meaning your blood sugar levels rise more slowly. Glycemic load (GL) is another term to describe how a carbohydrate food will affect your blood sugar. This measure takes into account both the

GI and the amount of carbohydrate available in the food. For example, pasta has a lower GI than watermelon, yet pasta has more carbs. So, if you eat similar amounts of either, it is the pasta that will have a greater affect on your blood sugar levels.

WHAT FOODS HAVE A HIGH GI?

Sugary and highly processed carbs typically have a high GI. Some consider these high-indexed foods as 'empty calories' since our body digests them so rapidly that we feel hungry soon after eating them. As a result, we continue eating, often choosing foods high in sugar to reach that sugar 'high' again. However, there are times when foods with a high GI come in handy – such as before a workout to give you a boost. Just keep in mind that the energy boost you feel will be short-lived.

WHAT FOODS HAVE A LOW GI?

Natural foods like most fruit, vegetables and whole grains like oats tend to have a low GI. These low GI foods are broken down more slowly and cause a more gradual rise in blood sugar levels.

So is the glycemic index the secret to optimal health? Only within the context of a balanced diet!

Just because a food has a high GI it does not necessarily mean it's not good for you. While low GI foods may appear to be healthiest, it's so important to appreciate their nutritional content first. It's also important to understand that foods that contain or are cooked with fat and protein slow down the release of carbohydrate, therefore lowering their overall GI. For example, potatoes and rice both have a high GI yet are nutritious and should be considered as part of a balanced diet. Pizza, crisps and chips all have a low GI but we all know they shouldn't be consumed every day. This example clearly shows that if you only eat foods with a low GI, you may find your diet is unbalanced. Another good example is agave syrup; it is marketed as healthy because it has a low GI but it is extremely high in sugar.

Carbs are an important part of a healthy balanced diet. Just try to include more of the starchy carbs that are high in fibre, such as wholegrain rice, pasta and bread, potatoes, quinoa, beans and lentils and eat fewer of the high-sugar varieties.

EATING THE RIGHT CARBS

If you have health problems like metabolic syndrome and/or type 2 diabetes, then you are more likely to be insulin resistant. In this case, reducing your portion of carbs can have clear benefits as you won't be requiring as much insulin. However, if you are generally healthy and are simply looking to optimise your diet and stay healthy, then there is absolutely no reason for you to avoid carbs. Ultimately, if you have any health condition such as diabetes, always consult your GP before making any dietary changes.

Many carb-containing foods are in fact very healthy, such as fruits and vegetables that provide a variety of nutrients. As a general rule, carbohydrates that are in their natural, fibre-rich form – complex carbs – are going to be good for you, whereas those that have been stripped of their fibre – simple carbs – are not going to do you any favours. If it's a whole, natural food then it's probably healthy for most people, no matter the carbohydrate content.

CARBS TO INCLUDE MORE OF IN YOUR DIET:	CARBS TO INCLUDE LESS OF IN YOUR DIET:
Brown rice	Chips and crisps
Buckwheat	Chocolate – usually high in sugar although opting for good-quality dark chocolate with a high cocoa solids percentage is a better choice
Fruits	
Legumes e.g. lentils, beans and peas	Fruit juices – these have similar effects as sugar-sweetened drinks as they lack the natural fibre within the whole fruit
Oats	
Quinoa	Ice cream
Starchy vegetables e.g. sweet potato, beetroot and corn	Pastries
Wholegrain bread	Sugary drinks
	White bread

MY 4 RULES ON CARBS

1. Be carb-conscious
    There is definitely a case for reducing the amount of refined carbohydrates (like white bread and white pasta) in your diet, instead opting for complex carbohydrates (like wholegrain bread and rice) as they release energy more slowly. I find thinking about 'grains' rather than 'carbs' makes it far simpler to understand and remember.

2. Not all carbs are created equal
    We must not forget that carbohydrates are an important source of fuel for your brain and body. Complex carbohydrates are a good source of vitamins and fibre, all helping your digestive system to stay healthy and keeping your blood sugar levels steady. They contain all sorts of micronutrients that help to slowly release the energy from food, keeping you fuller for longer too. Good, wholesome, starchy carbohydrates include wholegrain pasta, sweet potatoes, wholegrain rice and quinoa. Refined carbohydrate foods like pastries and white bread are usually lacking in essential nutrients.

3. Carbs make you happy
    Our brains use the glucose found in carbohydrates as fuel. If you've ever been on a strict diet regime avoiding carbohydrates you'll know that it can be hard to concentrate and you often experience severe mood swings. It's because carbs play an important role in creating serotonin (your happy hormone) in the brain.

4. Cutting carbs out completely is unsustainable
    Although some people experience initial weight loss from a no-carbohydrate diet, most can't maintain it. A balanced diet is what we should all be aiming for and if you're looking for weight loss, portion control and a bit of extra physical activity will give you better results.

NEVER BE WITHOUT PROTEIN

Protein is essential. It is so much more than simply food for your muscles: every single cell in our body contains protein. It also plays a key role in maintaining your mood, liver function, immunity, kidney health, hormone balance and adrenal function. However, thanks to images of bodybuilders chugging down post-workout protein shakes promising quick muscle gain, there is a stigma that protein makes us bulky, heavy and unhealthy. In fact, protein can aid fat burning and help weight loss alongside a healthy diet.[1] As you lose weight, your body may lose both fat and muscle, so having adequate protein coming from your diet fuels fat burning while preserving your lean muscle mass.

WHAT IS PROTEIN?

When eaten, protein is broken down into amino acids, otherwise known as the building blocks of protein. We need these amino acids for almost every metabolic process in the body. However, different proteins can vary greatly in the types of amino acids they contain. There are about 20 different types of amino acids, of which nine are collectively referred to as essential amino acids. Amino acids can only be supplied by the foods we eat, as our bodies cannot produce them naturally.

Amino acids can be thought of like letters of the alphabet. While we combine letters in different orders to make words, each combination of amino acid will create a different structure with thousands of possible combinations. Although it's not necessary to eat essential amino acids with every meal, just be aware your body requires a variety of protein sources to give you an adequate amount every day.

Complete protein sources
Complete proteins are those that contain all nine essential amino acids in sufficient quantities. They are typically from animal sources, but a few plant sources are also considered complete.

ANIMAL	PLANT-BASED
Dairy products (milk, yoghurt, whey)	Hemp
Eggs	Quinoa
Fish	Soya
Meat	

Incomplete sources

Incomplete proteins are other plant-based sources of protein that don't contain all nine essential amino acids, or don't have sufficient quantities of them to meet the body's daily requirements. Just because these are incomplete doesn't make them inferior though. They just need to be combined with other plant proteins to ensure you get the right balance of essential amino acids in your diet every day. In the right combination, they can make a complete amino acid profile – these pairings are known as complementary proteins. For this reason, vegans and vegetarians are often advised to eat a wide variety of protein-rich and fortified foods to ensure they consume all the nine essential amino acids each day.

◊ Nuts and seeds
◊ Legumes (e.g. lentils, beans and peas)
◊ Grains
◊ Vegetables

Ways to combine incomplete protein sources to create complete profiles
◊ Oats and nuts
◊ Brown rice and black beans
◊ Peanut butter on wholegrain bread

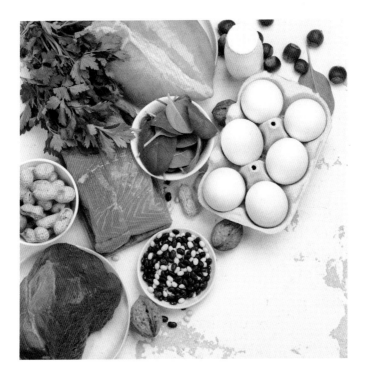

HOW MUCH PROTEIN DO WE NEED?

If you speak to different experts you will most likely get different answers to this question. However, they will all agree that, for the most part, it depends on your level of physical activity, your gender and your age. It is important to remember that protein should be about quality not quantity and that we each require different amounts.

If you have a physically demanding job, you walk a lot, run, swim or do any sort of exercise, then you need more protein. Adults are advised to eat 0.75g of protein per kilogram of bodyweight per day, based on the UK government Reference Nutrient Intake (RNI). So, if you weigh 70kg (11 stone), you should eat a minimum of 52.5g of protein a day.[2] Elderly people need significantly more protein, up to 50 per cent more than the recommended daily intake; this is because as we grow older, our bodies becomes less efficient at using protein, so eating more will make it more likely to meet the daily requirements.

Based on average weights and activity levels, men should aim to eat 55g and women 45g of protein daily. That's about 2 palm-sized portions of meat, fish, tofu, nuts or pulses. For those men and women who are particularly active, consuming at least 1g of protein per kg of weight is a sensible measure.

Most people in the Western world are eating enough protein to prevent deficiency, but there are some who would do better with a much higher protein intake. Numerous studies demonstrate that a high-protein diet has major benefits for your health. Here are five evidence-based reasons to eat more protein:

1. Protein can reduce appetite and hunger levels
    Gram for gram, protein helps you feel more full than carbs and fats. This is largely due to protein reducing your levels of the hunger hormone ghrelin and boosting satiety-related hormones.[3]

2. Protein can increase muscle mass and strength
    Eating plenty of protein can help increase muscle mass and strength as well as reduce muscle loss when losing weight.[4]

3. Protein is good for your bones
    People who eat more protein tend to have better bone health as they grow older; they have a much lower risk of osteoporosis and fractures (see page 42 for more on bone health). This is especially important for women, who are at high risk of osteoporosis after menopause. Eating plenty of protein and staying active is a good way to help prevent this.[5]

4.   Protein can lower your blood pressure

High blood pressure is attributed to heart attacks, strokes and chronic kidney disease. A higher protein intake has been shown to lower blood pressure as well as reduced LDL cholesterol and triglycerides (see page 37 for more on cholesterol).[6,7]

5.   Protein can help you keep fit as you get older

One of the consequences of ageing is that your muscles shrink. This is referred to as age-related disease sarcopenia and is one of the main causes of frailty and fractures. Given protein forms the main building blocks of the body's tissues and organs, eating more protein after injury can help speed up recovery or daily performance.[8]

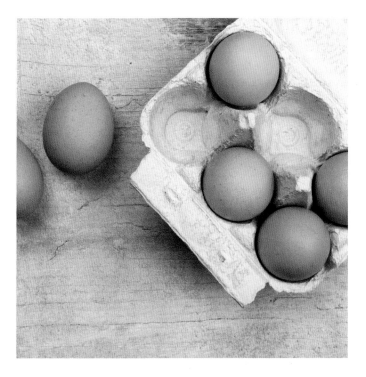

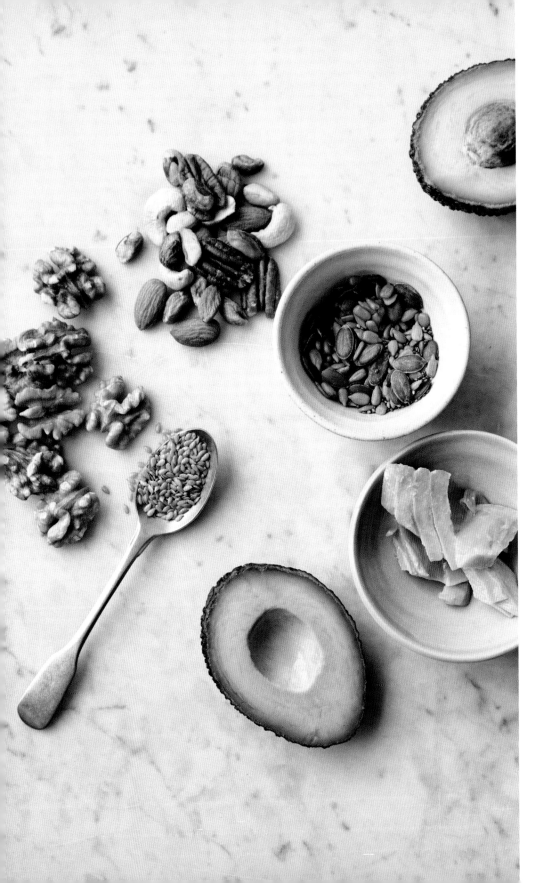

WHERE ARE YOUR HEALTHY FATS?

Fats are absolutely essential for a healthy lifestyle and I encourage you all to include a portion at every single meal. However, it is important to be conscious of portion sizes given that fats are the most energy-dense of all the macronutrients i.e. more calories per gram than protein and carbs.

THE DIFFERENT TYPES OF FAT

There are three key types of fat, each unique in their chemical structure: saturated fats, unsaturated fats and trans fats. Fats with a single-bond structure are saturated, while fats with a double-bonded structure are unsaturated. The type of bond affects how each type of fat works inside our bodies and determines their impact on our health. Most foods containing fat naturally contain a mixture of the different types of fat, so it is difficult to totally exclude one group in favour of another. However, we should all be aiming to cut out trans fats, cut down on saturated fats and increase mono and polyunsaturated fats, particularly omega-3.

Saturated fats

These come mainly from animal sources and tend to be solid at room temperature – for example, butter. They are very stable at high temperatures and far less likely to be damaged during cooking than polyunsaturated fats, which is why they have traditionally been used in cake recipes. Saturated fats are the least healthy fats and the latest Cochrane Review found that by reducing the consumption of saturated fat, it decreased the incidence of heart disease by 17%.[9] We still eat too much saturated fat in the UK and should still be trying to reduce this amount. However, as part of a balanced healthy diet we can have up to 11% of our total energy intake from saturated fat.

Unsaturated fats

Monounsaturated fatty acids (MUFAs) are typically liquid at room temperature and are fairly stable for cooking purposes. The most common MUFA is oleic acid, which is present in olive oil in high amounts. Excellent sources of this healthy fat can be found in avocados, nuts, seeds, fish oils and nut oils. Monounsaturated fats are linked to several health benefits, including a reduced risk of serious diseases such as heart disease and diabetes.[10]

Polyunsaturated fatty acids (PUFAs) are found in oily fish, walnuts, flaxseeds and vegetable oils. These include omega-3 and omega-6 fats. Studies have found that omega-3 fats have benefits for inflammation (see overleaf), heart disease, diabetes, depression and other health conditions.[11] Omega-6 fats on the other hand have been found to be detrimental to our health – put simply, a diet high in omega-6 but low in omega-3 is believed to increase inflammation.[12] So it is a good idea to eat plenty of omega-3 (such as from fatty fish), but most people would also do well to reduce their omega-6 consumption.[13]

Ultimately we need to be really looking at increasing our Omega-3 fats, as these are usually consumed in much smaller amounts and found in less commonly consumed foods such as oily fish, flaxseed and walnuts. Aiming to reduce saturated fats and trans fats and increase the healthy mono and poly unsaturated fats (Omega-3) will put us all in good stead.

What is inflammation?

Inflammation is essential for our survival, helping us protect our bodies from infection and injury, but it can also cause severe damage and contribute to disease when the inflammatory response is excessive. In fact, excess inflammation may be one of the leading drivers of the most serious diseases today, including heart disease, metabolic syndrome, diabetes, arthritis, Alzheimer's and many types of cancer.

Trans fats

Trans fats are well and truly on the 'completely avoid' list. Most are produced by adding hydrogen to unsaturated fats to create a product that functions in a similar way to saturated fat. Ingredient labels often list them as 'partially hydrogenated' fats. They are added, for example, to margarine and other heavily processed spreads to ensure the texture and flavour are preserved as well as to give the product an increased shelf life. Although small amounts of trans fats do occur naturally in dairy and other animal foods, there is nothing natural about the trans fats used in processed foods. Trans fats are now not such a big problem in the UK as the manufacturing industry has been reducing their use over the years, in line with government healthy eating guidelines, but it is important to be aware that consuming trans fats can lead to a number of health problems. Artificial trans fats are linked to inflammation, unhealthy cholesterol levels, impaired artery function, insulin resistance and excess belly fat.[14]

THE BENEFITS OF FATS

◊ Energy Fat is an excellent energy source. It provides 9 calories per gram, whereas protein and carbs each provide 4 calories per gram.

◊ Hormone function Fat plays a major role in the production of hormones.[15]

◊ Brain function Fat intake is important for cognition and can have a positive impact on mood. It can stimulate the growth of new brain cells and improve memory too.[16]

◊ **Absorption** of fat-soluble vitamins – vitamins A, D, E and K. Without fat, these important nutrients cannot be absorbed.

◊ **Flavour and fullness** Adding fat to foods makes them tastier and more satisfying. So, drizzle your salad with a teaspoon of olive oil as it might stop you reaching for the snacks later.

◊ **Omega-3** This is crucial for our health, hormones, immune system, blood clotting and cellular growth. Try to have up to two portions of oily fish every week and enjoy a variety of nuts and seeds in small quantities.

WHAT'S THE DEAL WITH CHOLESTEROL?

Cholesterol is produced in the liver and has managed to get itself a rather bad name, even though it's a perfectly natural fat-like substance.

In order for cholesterol to be carried in your bloodstream, your liver coats it in proteins. The tiny balls of fat that are produced are called lipoproteins and this is what is usually being referred to when we mention cholesterol. There are two main types: high-density lipoproteins (HDL) and low-density lipoproteins (LDL), known as the 'good' and 'bad' cholesterols respectively.

Ultimately, you want to aim to have a high level of HDL and a low level of LDL. The problem with checking your total cholesterol (HDL + LDL) is that you don't know the ratio of good to bad. I personally have high cholesterol levels and I used to be very concerned about this until I was tested for both and found I have a high protective amount of HDL.

Follow these tips to increase your HDL and reduce your LDL:

Eat olive oil
Olive oil with a high polyphenol content has been shown to increase HDL levels in healthy people, the elderly and individuals with high cholesterol.[17]

Eat avocados
Avocados contain monounsaturated fatty acids and fibre, two heart-healthy and cholesterol-lowering nutrients.

Stop smoking
Quitting smoking can increase HDL levels, improve HDL function and help protect heart health.

Eat purple

Consuming purple fruits and vegetables that are rich in anthocyanins may help increase HDL cholesterol levels.[18]

Eat oily fish

Eating fatty fish several times a week may help increase HDL cholesterol levels and provide other benefits to heart health.[19]

Exercise

Even low-intensity exercising several times per week can help raise HDL cholesterol and enhance its anti-inflammatory and antioxidant effects.[20]

Limit trans fats

Artificial trans fats have been shown to lower HDL levels and increase inflammation, compared to other fats.

Eat whole grains

Whole grains are linked to a lower risk of heart disease. Oats and barley contain beta-glucan, a soluble fibre that is very effective at lowering LDL cholesterol.[21]

Eat nuts

Nuts are rich in cholesterol-lowering fats and fibre, as well as minerals that are linked to improved heart health.[22]

Eat legumes

Legumes like beans, peas and lentils can help lower LDL levels and are a good source of plant-based proteins.[23]

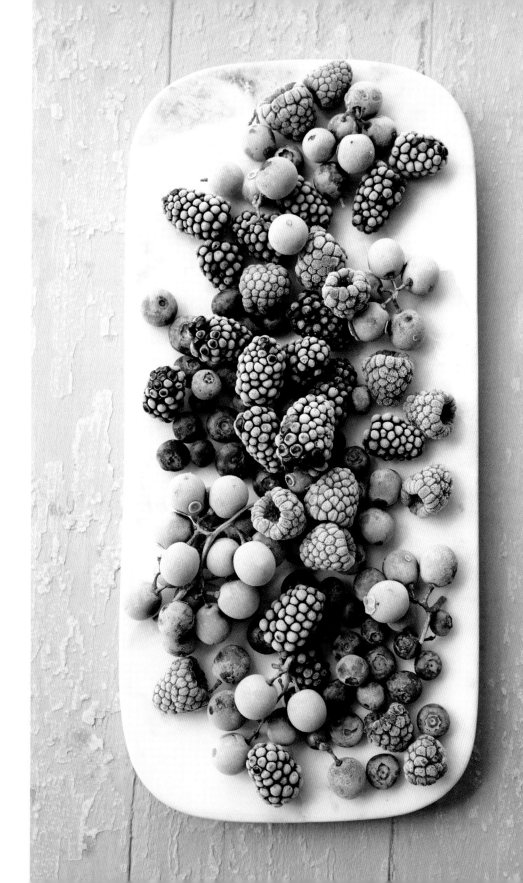

MICRONUTRIENTS

Micronutrients are the vitamins and minerals we need to ensure optimal health and prevent nutritional deficiencies. Getting a variety of nutrition and colour in our diets is key. All of the vitamins and minerals are 'essential' nutrients, meaning you can only get them from your diet. The daily requirement of each micronutrient varies between individuals but if you eat a healthy balanced diet that includes both plants and animals, then you should be getting all of the micronutrients your body needs without taking a supplement. If you don't eat animal products, just be aware of potential nutritional deficiencies. However, a well balanced diet should still provide the essential nutrients you need; see a registered nutritionist or dietitian if you wish to enhance it. These micronutrients enable the body to produce enzymes and hormones and are required for optimal growth and development. Although their required amounts are small, the consequences of their absence can be severe. When it comes to nutrition, sometimes you have to think small to get big results. The World Health Organization suggests that micronutrient deficiency represents some of the most common and widespread nutritional disorders in the world.

It is also important to note that vitamins are available in two forms: water-soluble and fat-soluble. Water-soluble vitamins are easily lost through bodily fluids and must be replaced each day. These include the B vitamins and vitamin C. Fat-soluble vitamins tend to accumulate within the body and are not needed on a daily basis. These include vitamins A, D, E and K.

Calcium
Calcium is an important structural component of bones and teeth, as well as a key mineral for your heart, muscles and nervous system.
Sources include milk, yoghurt, spinach and sardines (if you eat their bones).

Iodine
An essential mineral for normal thyroid function and the production of thyroid hormones. Thyroid hormones are involved in many processes in the body, such as growth, brain development and bone maintenance. They also regulate the metabolic rate. Iodine deficiency is one of the most common nutrient deficiencies in the world. It affects nearly one-third of the world's population.
Sources include fish, dairy and eggs.

Iron
Iron deficiency is the most common in the world, and the only one prevalent in developed countries. Over 30 per cent of the world's population suffers from anaemia, which lowers the ability of the blood to carry oxygen. Iron has many other benefits, including improved immune and brain function.
Sources include shellfish, broccoli, red meat and tofu.

Magnesium

Magnesium plays a role in over 600 cellular processes, including energy production, nervous system function and muscle contraction.

Sources include avocados, nuts and leafy greens.

Potassium

Potassium is important for blood pressure control, fluid balance and muscles and nerve function.

Sources include bananas, spinach, potatoes and apricots.

Vitamins A and E

These are powerful antioxidants, helping protect cells from free radicals and ageing. Vitamin A contributes to cell renewal and repair; vitamin E reduces the effects of skin ageing and the risk of skin cancer. (NOTE: reduce vitamin A during pregnancy, as in excess it may be harmful to the baby.)

Sources of vitamin A include carrots and sweet potatoes. Sources of vitamin E include almonds and avocados.

Vitamin B12 and Folate

Your DNA, red blood cells and the metabolism of each cell inside your body need these vitamins. B12 is necessary for a healthy nervous system while folate plays a role in brain and spinal chord development in unborn babies, which is why all pregnant women or women trying to conceive are advised to take a folate supplement.

B12 is only found in animal products, such as eggs, meat or fish or fortified plant foods. If you are vegan, I highly advise reviewing whether you are getting enough.

Vitamin C

This wonderful antioxidant is hailed as the cure to colds and flu because it contributes to healing. It also maintains healthy skin, blood vessels and cartilage and plays a role in the production of collagen, which maintains our skin's elasticity and strength.

Sources include oranges, peppers, broccoli and bananas.

Vitamin D

Vitamin D is special as it is made inside your body after the skin has been exposed to sunlight. Low levels have been linked to depression and a variety of mood disorders. The UK Government now recommends supplementing with vitamin D in the winter months.

Sources include fortified foods (select milks and cereals), oily fish with bones, yoghurt and egg yolks.

Zinc

Zinc supports our immune system, hormone production and fertility. It is also beneficial for skin as it can help reduce inflammation, helps wound healing and protect us against UV damage from the sun.

Sources include shellfish, red meat, eggs and chickpeas.

BONE HEALTH

An area that is often overlooked is our skeleton. Most health and fitness goals tend to be aesthetic or focussing solely on the amount of muscle and fat in our bodies. We often overlook our physical structure, the building blocks of our very existence. Osteoporosis in on the rise and is a crippling disease affecting thousands of women and men every year. This is not just a case of brittle bones; osteoporosis can kill. I hate to use such drastic language but we all need to be aware of how serious this condition can be.

Perhaps the biggest worry is that this is known as a 'silent' disease. Often you don't notice anything until it's too late and symptoms when presented often worsen quickly – a fracture can occur from just a small bump or minor accident.

I especially want to raise this issue with young women as I see a lot of concerning cases in my clinic. We don't reach peak bone density (or peak bone mass) until around the age of 25 to 30, at which point our bones have reached their maximum strength. More often than not, young people are not reaching this peak because of lifestyle factors such as smoking, poor diet, eating disorders and lack of exercise. This is why it's so important to start looking after our bodies sooner rather than later.

There is so much more to bone health than just drinking milk and eating dairy products. Every single type of food we eat significantly affects our bones. Magnesium (found in avocados, dark leafy greens and nuts – almonds, cashews and brazil nuts especially) is the most abundant mineral in our bones after calcium. We need vitamin D to aid both calcium and magnesium absorption, and to absorb vitamin D you need healthy fats. So you see, calcium is not the only answer – a whole array of vitamins and minerals is required for healthy bones.

Having said that, it is crucial we get enough calcium in our diets to build strong bones, teeth and even regulate muscle contractions inside our body, including our heartbeat! In the UK the current guidelines for calcium are, per day:

Men and women: 700mg

Breastfeeding women: 1,250mg

Teenage boys: 1,000mg daily

Teenage girls: 800mg

Younger children: 350–525mg

CALCIUM-RICH FOODS

FOOD	CALCIUM PER 100mg
Cheddar cheese	271
Tofu	162
Figs	145
Whole eggs	139
Milk	119
Hazelnuts	113
Trout	86
Miso	65
Chickpeas	49
Broccoli	48

The above list gives you a rough idea of what calcium-rich foods you should be looking to include in your diet, but there are many more foods out there to choose from. Try to think about the sources you are choosing at each meal. For example, 200g of cooked kale contains the same amount of calcium as 225ml of milk. Tinned whole sardines contain more calcium weight for weight than milk – and with the added benefit of omega-3 (see Where are Your Healthy Fats?, page 35).

FIBRE

A simple explanation of dietary fibre is food that cannot be digested. However, this doesn't give fibre the credit it is due. There are different types of fibre, each having different effects on our body and health and all of them providing numerous health benefits. Fibre helps us stay fuller for longer, keeps our digestion healthy and reduces the likelihood of weight gain.

Including plenty of fibre in your diet has been proven to actively work towards lowering your risk of heart disease, diabetes, weight gain and even some cancers. Most people get on average 18g a day when you should be aiming for 30g a day. A food high in fibre is considered to have 6g of fibre per 100g, so do check the information on food labels when buying food.[24]

Fibre is classified by its solubility in water, with two types, both of which play a key role as part of a healthy balanced diet. Insoluble fibre doesn't dissolve in water and passes through us without being broken down. This can help push other food items through, preventing digestive problems. However, if you have diarrhoea then avoid insoluble fibre in the short term! Soluble fibre dissolves in water in our digestive system and has been linked to reducing cholesterol in the blood. Gradually increasing the amount of soluble fibre in the diet can help with constipation as it can help soften the stools, making them easier to pass through.

Top sources of insoluble fibre:

◊ Wholegrain bread
◊ Bran
◊ Some cereals e.g. All Bran
◊ Nuts and seeds

Top sources of soluble fibre:

◊ Oats (try my porridge on pages 120–1)
◊ Fruit (e.g. bananas, apples)
◊ Root vegetables
◊ Flaxseeds

WARNING: Never suddenly alter your diet without supervision; suddenly increasing fibre can cause problems, such as bloating and loose bowel movements just as suddenly reducing it can cause harm. Try to drink 2 litres of water a day.

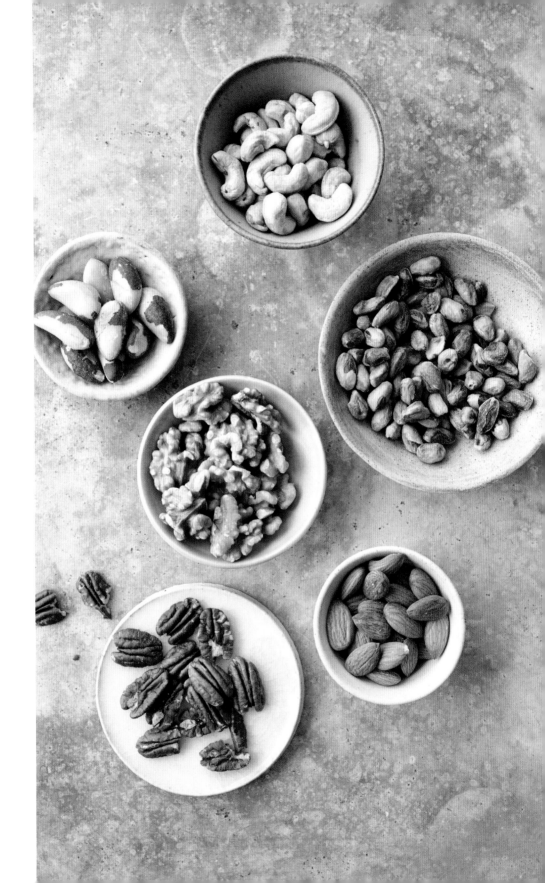

A HEALTHY GUT

You could be eating the healthiest diet in the world but if it's not being absorbed effectively then it's all to no avail. Our digestion is far from a simple process; it involves a series of hormonal signals working throughout the gut and our nervous system. Most evidence suggests that it takes up to 20 minutes for our brain to acknowledge when we are feeling full, which explains why when someone eats too quickly, they can eat a lot more than they really need.

Many companies slip in the 'friendly bacteria' claim when selling certain products but this actually has scientific basis to it. A lot of our immunity is dependent upon our gut and the microbes that live within it. Very few gut bacteria live in the small intestine; they tend to be found towards the end of the digestive process. It is therefore essential for our health that the equilibrium in the gut remains this way. If you are suffering from symptoms such as bloating, joint pain or repeated gastrointestinal infections then you may have a bacterial overgrowth or bacteria may have travelled 'the wrong way' up the small intestine.[25]

The bacteria inside our gut are full of useful nutrition but we are unable to re-absorb them (like some creatures that eat their own faeces), so it's important to keep topping up our bacteria with food. This is why prebiotics and probiotics are so important for a happy tummy and our overall health. However, they play different roles:

Probiotics are live bacteria found in certain foods or supplements. They can provide numerous health benefits. Fermented foods, such as yoghurt, sauerkraut, kimchi and other pickled ingredients are good sources.

Prebiotics are substances that come from types of foods (mostly fibre) that humans can't digest. They are a source of food for the beneficial bacteria in your gut and you needn't look far for them – vegetables, fruit and legumes all contain prebiotic fibre, although some contain more than others such as, onions, garlic, bananas and beans.

Eating balanced amounts of both probiotics and prebiotics can help ensure that you have the right balance of these bacteria, which should improve your health.

MY TOP 5 BACTERIA-FRIENDLY (PROBIOTIC) FOODS

Kefir

Kefir is a fermented probiotic milk drink. It is made by adding kefir grains to cow's or goat's milk. Kefir grains are not cereal grains, but rather cultures of lactic acid bacteria and yeast. Kefir contains several major strains of friendly bacteria and yeast, making it a diverse and potent probiotic. Like yoghurt, kefir is generally well tolerated by people who are lactose intolerant.

Sauerkraut

Sauerkraut is finely shredded cabbage that has been fermented by lactic acid bacteria. Added to its probiotic qualities, sauerkraut is rich in fibre, as well as vitamins B, C and K. It is also high in sodium and contains iron, manganese and the antioxidants important for eye health. Always choose unpasteurised sauerkraut as pasteurisation kills the live and active bacteria. One of the oldest traditional foods, it is popular in many countries, especially in Europe.

Yoghurt

Yoghurt is made from milk fermented by friendly bacteria, mainly lactic acid bacteria and bifidobacteria. Yoghurt may be better than milk for people with lactose intolerance because the bacteria turn some of the lactose into lactic acid, which is what gives yoghurt its sour taste. However, keep in mind that not all yoghurt contains live probiotics. In some cases, the live bacteria have been killed during processing. Choose yoghurt with active or live cultures and always read the label – many low-fat or fat-free yoghurts are often loaded with sugar.

Kimchi

Kimchi is a fermented, spicy Korean side dish. Cabbage is usually the main ingredient, but it can also be made from other vegetables. Kimchi contains the lactic acid bacteria lactobacillus kimchii, as well as other lactic acid bacteria. Kimchi made from cabbage is high in some vitamins and minerals, including vitamin K, riboflavin (vitamin B2) and iron.

Kombucha

Kombucha is a black or green tea drink fermented by a friendly colony of bacteria and yeast. It is consumed in many parts of the world, especially Asia. There are many claims about the health effects of kombucha but high-quality evidence is lacking. However, as kombucha is fermented with bacteria and yeast, it is likely to have health benefits related to its probiotic properties.

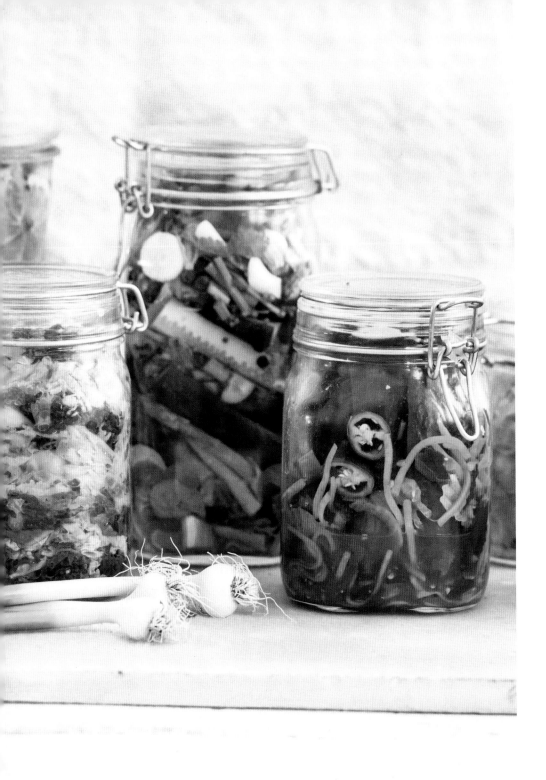

WEIGHT AND THE GUT

Certain types of food are only broken down as a direct result of the action of our gut microbes; in fact, around 10 per cent of the food we eat is broken down entirely by our bacteria. This is why our weight is not always affected by the quantity of food we eat but the type of food as well – it's the bacteria in your gut that are being fed as well so if you feed it food it likes, it will use it well.

Some recent studies suggest that:

◊   Bacteria affect our appetite. When we eat food our bacteria likes, we increase our satiety-signal transmitters, meaning we are less likely to reach for more food.

◊   Bacteria make us feel good when we get a decent source of food by influencing our happy signals in our brain.

◊   Bacteria love the type of food that reach them relatively undigested (prebiotic foods).

◊   We are all unique and the microbes that live in our gut can affect how much energy we take from food; basically some of us are more prone to weight gain than others even when eating the same amount of food.

◊   Bacteria may also have an effect on our thyroid gland, causing it to produce fewer hormones and affecting the speed at which we burn fat.

Ultimately, we need to look at our nutrition in a bigger way. Now we know about the existence of gut bacteria, we can ensure we have a good level of gut bacteria and slowly build up our intake of prebiotic foods. From this we will then be re-training the signals inside our body and re-aligning a wonderful system that is in place already.

DRINK MORE

I advise everyone to drink more water every day. Too many of us are simply not drinking enough, but how much water should you drink every day? Estimates report the average Briton drinks less than 1 glass of water a day, preferring instead to take in fluids in the form of sugary drinks, tea, coffee and juices.

Our bodies are comprised largely of water so it's understandable that every function inside our body depends on it to do its job well. Cells, organs and tissues all need water and it's absolutely essential that we drink enough. And when we have enough water we become more efficient at losing it too, through sweating and urination. This is crucial to eradicate toxins from the body and prevent us from becoming unwell.

Most of us should aim to drink 2 litres of water every day. Getting a nice (BPA free) reusable water bottle will help you keep track of your daily water intake and remember, if you sweat a lot you need to replenish that lost water. Some say that when we feel thirsty we have already lost 1% of the total amount of water in our body. Here are some reasons we should all drink more water:

Hungry or thirsty?
Sometimes we think we are hungry, when actually we are thirsty.

Be less cranky
Dehydration affects your mood, making you grumpy. Drinking more water will help you think more clearly and be happier, making you better prepared for regular healthy eating.

Perform better
Water is essential for the proper circulation of nutrients in the body. Water serves as the body's transportation system; when we are dehydrated things just can't get around as well as they should. Water comprises 75 per cent of our muscle tissue so proper hydration contributes to increased mental and physical performance. Dehydration leads to weakness and fatigue.

Flush out bad bacteria
Our digestive system needs water to function properly. If we don't drink water, we don't flush out waste and it collects in our body, causing a myriad of problems.

Keep your bowels regular
A major part of constipation is often not consuming enough fluid. If you suffer from constipation, try to increase the overall fluids you are consuming.

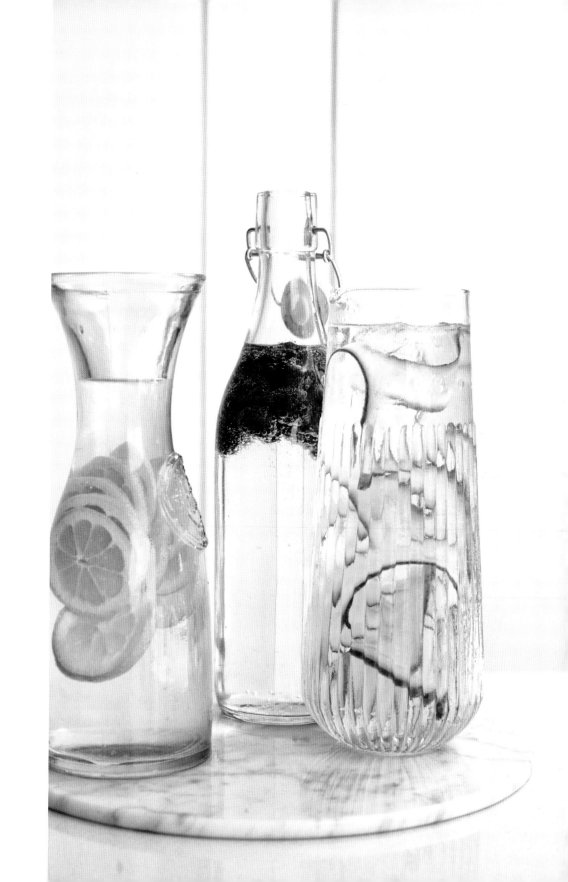

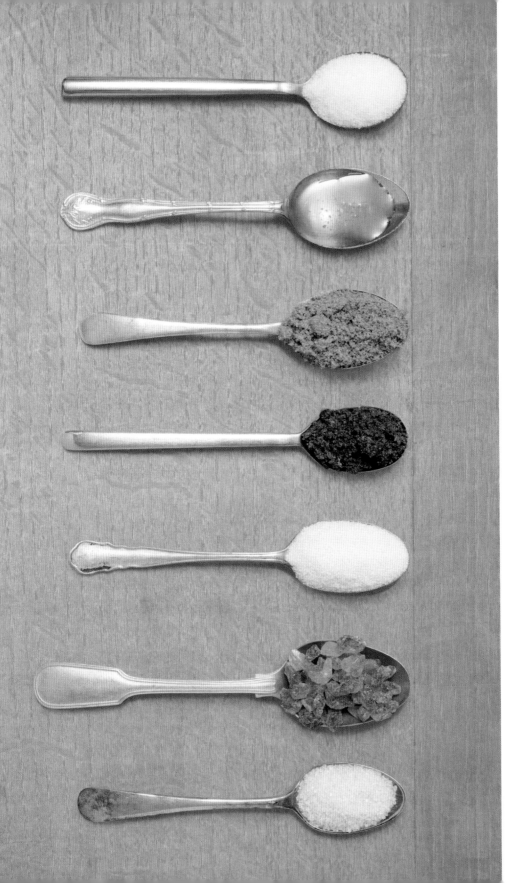

SUGAR

The role that refined sugar plays in our health is simple: it's of zero value to us nutritionally. In order to understand what is so bad about sugar, you need to understand what it is made of. Sugar (the white stuff) is composed of two molecules, glucose and fructose. Glucose is found in nearly all carbohydrates and fructose is found in fruit and some vegetables. While they have identical chemical formulas and weigh the same, our body sees them completely differently.

Ultimately, every cell in the body can make use of glucose, while the liver is the only organ that can metabolise fructose in significant amounts. A diet high in fructose will mean the liver becomes overloaded. Athletes or highly active individuals can eat quite a bit of fructose without problems, because their livers will turn the fructose into glycogen – a storage form of glucose in the liver. However, when someone's liver is already full of glycogen (which is true of most people), the fructose may be turned into fat.

There is countless research demonstrating that sugar, more than any other ingredient, may be driving some of the world's most deadly conditions, including heart disease, diabetes and cancer. Previously, the public health message has been to eat less saturated fat. Removing fat from foods makes them less tasty so food companies added significant amounts of sugar to compensate. People started eating huge amounts of added sugars, without even realising it.

Research suggests that today we're eating about 22 teaspoons of added sugar per day, or 355 calories, amounting to 32kg per year.[26] Unfortunately, people don't appreciate how much sugar they're actually eating. They aren't pouring 22 teaspoons of sugar into drinks, they're getting it from heavily processed foods. Frustratingly, food manufacturers often use confusing terms for sugar to hide the true amount of sugar in their foods. Instead of reaching for sugary drinks, try infusing water with fresh fruit – my favourite is mint, lemon and lime or mixed berries. And, you can eat the fruit afterwards just like you would do after a Pimm's, or is that just me?!

Confusingly, some foods that are considered healthy, such as fruit, also have high levels of sugar. This doesn't mean you should fear the likes of fruit and vegetables; fruit contains lots of water, as well as essential vitamins and minerals. There are, however, a few instances where minimising fruit might be a good idea, including if you are diabetic. However, for otherwise healthy people, there is no proven reason to avoid natural, whole fruit. The harmful effects of excess fructose only arise from added sugars. They do not apply to moderate consumption of fruit and vegetables.

Tip: Aim to reduce sugars in your diet. The NHS recommends food with less than 5g of total sugars per 100g.

COUNTING CALORIES

As discussed in My Philosophy (see page 12) calories are an important guide in terms of the energy food provides, but it's not as simple as just that. A calorie is effectively the energy required to heat a kilogram of water by 1°C.

Calories have proven useful in estimating the food requirements of large populations, such as developing standardised rations for troops or organising humanitarian relief. In times of shortage the calorie makes it easier to assign food resources efficiently. But as a guide to eating well they prove a mixed blessing.

While many people treat calorie estimates as concrete figures, they are at best approximations that do not take into account individual differences in food absorption, metabolism or the effects of cooking on increasing food's digestibility.

I have seen in my clinical work that when people feel they should maintain a minimal calorific intake at all costs, they can very quickly disregard the social and physical pleasures and traditions associated with eating – even disregarding their own personal preference. Counting calories can provide a sense of control for some dieters but it often ends up becoming all-consuming, resulting in a lonely, competitive dieting culture.

Rather than helping, being overly conscious of calories may make eating a confusing and perilous activity. I frequently convey my philosophy of nutrients over numbers (see page 16) in order to break free from the endless regimented counting. Calories aren't everything; not by any means. With every mouthful, we are affecting our hormones and brain, which govern when, what and how much we eat; it's not as simple as counting calories.

WARNING: The food industry has spent a lot of money trying to create low-calorie products that taste as good as their natural, higher-calorie counterparts. This does not make them healthier choices; often the item in question will have added extras.

STARVATION IS NOT THE ANSWER

In 1944, an experiment on the psychological and physiological effects of starvation known as the Minnesota Starvation Experiment changed the way we now look at calorie-controlled diets. The physical and psychological symptoms described were the result of semi-starvation, which consisted of consuming 1,570 calories a day. Rather worryingly is that this calorie amount is similar or even higher than many of the unsupervised diet plans prescribed across the Internet today (often ranging from 800–1,400 calories). The symptoms reported ring true with many of my clients who have embarked upon a restrictive diet and then fallen prey to binge eating behaviours, fatigue, obsession with food, irritability and bouts of depression. Please do not embark upon a very low-calorie diet unsupervised. Without guidance, it may damage your mind, body and soul in unimaginable ways.[27]

Some lessons we can take away from the Minnesota Starvation Study, or at least thoughts to consider, are:

◊ Starvation, whether voluntary or involuntary, is incredibly difficult emotionally and physically.

◊ Even healthy people, who are not inclined towards disordered eating behaviours, will become obsessed with food and eating when they are deprived of adequate nourishment.

◊ Anyone restricting their eating will likely feel fatigued and unable to concentrate, disrupting any routine.

◊ Bingeing may be the result of restrictive eating and not due to a lack of self-control or willpower.

◊ The effects of starvation are gender neutral. Although all subjects in the Minnesota study were male, the characteristics and symptoms of starvation are identical to those experienced by women in similar circumstances.

◊ It also demonstrates that the body is not simply 'reprogrammed' once weight loss has been achieved. The volunteers' experimental diet was unsuccessful in overriding the body's strong desire to reach its happy weight level.

A BALANCED PLATE

I refer to the balanced plate every single day. Life is too short to be counting calories but we do need to be aware of how to eat healthily – for life not just for weight loss. My balanced plate, which is based on the Mediterranean diet and the use of fat-soluble vitamins, will help you achieve optimum nutrition, be free from cravings and will satisfy your body's every need without using numbers to guide you.

Focus on eating real food, and by real food I mean whole foods – items that are natural and perfectly designed for our body, offerring true nourishment. Also, you are far less likely to overeat if you satisfy your body's demands – believe me, willpower has nothing to do with it; a lot of the time it is your body crying out for what it truly needs.

It's impossible to eat perfectly (whatever that means to you) all the time, so I suggest using my principles for a balanced plate as a guide whenever you can. On some days there may not be an abundance of green vegetables for lunch – that's ok, just try and use the next mealtime as an opportunity to add some more. On some days of the week you may not be particularly active and may not need a large carbohydrate portion, so it's absolutely fine to lower it. Take into account your daily energy requirements and, in doing so, you'll start listening to your body.

I tend to find a really simple and easy way of gauging the size of your plate can be to make use of your hands. This cannot be 100 per cent accurate but in social situations it is a great reminder ascertaining whether or not we are fuelling our bodies with too little, too much or just the right amount of nutrition. As a general rule for everyone, you can follow hand portion sizes.

A 1 palm of protein e.g. chicken and fish

B 1 handful of carbohydrate e.g. rice, oats, starchy vegetables and fruit

C 2 handfuls of non-starchy vegetables e.g. broccoli, spinach and peppers

D 1 thumb of healthy fats e.g. olive oil, butter, coconut oil and nut butter

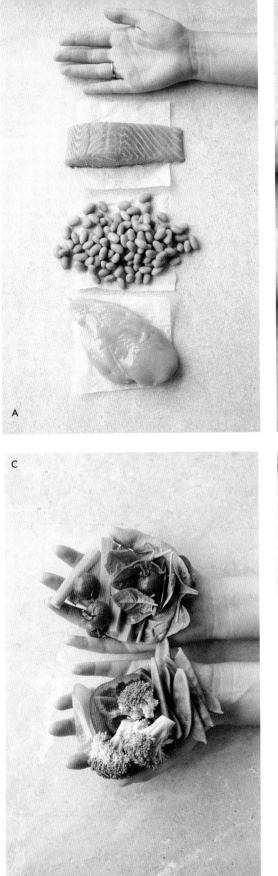

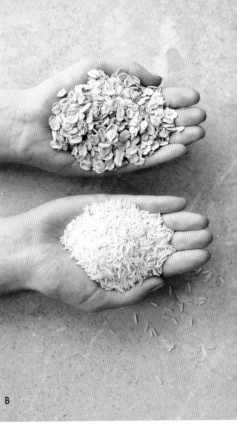

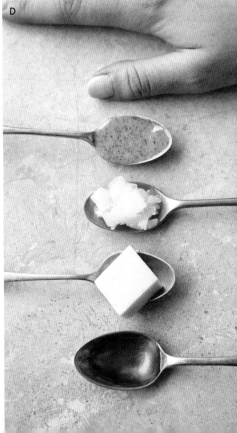

1 portion of protein (aim for 2 portions of oily fish a week and just 1 portion of red meat or processed meat a week)

1 portion of complex carbohydrate

1 large portion of non-starchy, fibrous vegetables

1 small portion of healthy fat

Occasional fruit as snacks (2–3 portions per day for a fibre and micronutrient boost)

HEALTHY FOODS TO INCLUDE ON YOUR PLATE

VEGETABLES	**Starchy:** Butternut squash, Sweet potatoes, White potatoes **Leafy and colourful:** Asparagus, Aubergine, Broccoli, Cauliflower, Courgettes, Green beans, Kale, Mushrooms, Onions, Pak choi, Peppers, Spinach, Tomatoes,
PROTEINS	Beef, Chicken, Eggs, Fish, Quorn, Tempeh, Tofu, Turkey
CARBOHYDRATES	Brown rice, Buckwheat, Oats, Quinoa, Rye bread, Spelt, Wholegrain
BEANS AND PULSES	Beans, Chickpeas, Lentils
HEALTHY FATS	Avocado, Coconut oil, Grass-fed butter, Nut butter, Nuts, Oily fish, Olive oil, Seeds, Tahini
DAIRY	Cottage cheese, Feta, Greek yoghurt, Halloumi, Milk, Unsweetened dairy-free fortified milk, Whey protein
FRUIT	Apples, Bananas, Berries, Cherries, Citrus, Kiwi, Melon, Pears, Peaches, Watermelon

MODERATION IS KEY

A realistic way of looking at life is that we cannot possibly be perfect all the time. Now go ahead and apply this to your nutrition too. Everyone harps on about 'balance'; have you truly found yours yet? Believe it or not, having the odd indulgence can be really good for you, just try to make sure it's not all the time. Your relationship with food and your body will only benefit from a relaxed approach. I tend to live by the 80/20 rule: I am 'healthy' 80 per cent of the time and then for the other 20 per cent I don't worry about it. For others the split can be 70/30 or 90/10 – whatever works for you. Forget about your friends and what the magazines say, do what you can achieve. (A Healthy Relationship with Food, page 18.)

BREAKING THE CYCLE

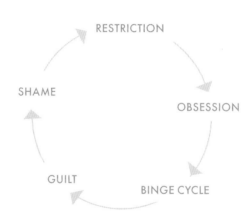

RESTRICTION

SHAME

OBSESSION

GUILT

BINGE CYCLE

If you ever find yourself stuck in the above cycle then think about the following:

1. Be prepared to work on yourself, your self-worth and self-esteem alongside your expectations and values. These all run deep in this type of cycle. Seek a professional such as a therapist who specialises in disordered eating.

2. Work on a food and mood diary and ensure you eat balanced meals (see page 56) three times a day with a couple of snacks if needed. Set yourself a small goal first of two consecutive days and just keep going – before you know it you'll be feeling more in control.

3. Remind yourself that your body needs fuel and food is your medicine. If your body is happy and receiving the nutrition it needs you are less likely to suffer from ill health.

4. Be kind to yourself; write down your logical thoughts as well as irrational ones in your food diary. You may be surprised to find you are bullying yourself with a nagging inner critic in your head. This is a sign some serious self-soothing or help in this area is required.

WARNING: If you believe you're suffering from an eating disorder or any form of disordered eating, I would encourage you to seek professional help at the earliest opportunity. Your GP will be your first point of contact as they can refer you to a registered health professional. Alternatively, you can seek private support. There is plenty of support out there.

ALCOHOL AND YOUR HEALTH

There is no denying that alcohol should be limited as part of a healthy diet. All too often I see alcohol associated with weight gain and poor mental clarity. Any positive claims from alcohol stem largely from studies using quality red wine and often on males over the age of 50. There is a lot of research investigating the powerful plant compounds in red wine and their health benefits, including reduced inflammation, lower risk of heart disease and extended lifespan. As with all good things, moderation is key, so keep an eye on your units.

The idea of counting alcohol units in the UK was first introduced in 1987. Units are a simple way of expressing the quantity of pure alcohol in a drink. One unit contains 10ml or 8g of pure alcohol, which is roughly the amount of alcohol the average adult can process in an hour. The number of units in a drink varies enormously, depending on the size of the drink, as well as its alcohol strength.

◊ A small shot of spirits (50ml) contains 1 unit
◊ A small glass of wine (125ml) contains 1.5 units
◊ A pint of low-strength lager has just over 2 units
◊ A large glass of wine (250ml) contains 3 units
◊ A pint of beer contains 3 units

Men and women are advised not to drink more than 14 units a week. Choose your alcohol wisely and remember that alcohol can be addictive and excessive consumption can cause a whole host of health issues.

ALCOHOL AND WEIGHT GAIN

There is an undeniable link between alcohol and weight gain so if you are looking to lose weight, learn to enjoy and savour one drink and then stop there. If you know you can't stop at one then you may need to re-consider your drinking habits. Try these simple tips:

◊ Keep sipping water, alternating drinks of alcohol and water.

◊ Don't drink on an empty stomach, try and always eat a meal beforehand. And avoid ordering takeaway food after drinking: you will always be tempted to order the unhealthiest foods.

◊ Try cutting down with a friend or partner as you'll be more likely to stick to it and break bad habits.

◊ Try not to drink alcohol with your meal.

◊ If you love your glass of wine, make it go further by adding some soda water to make a spritzer.

◊ If spirits are your thing, be wary as many can be high in sugar when combined with mixers. Consider vodka, lime and soda for a lighter option.

PHYSICAL ACTIVITY

Exercise is any movement that makes your muscles work and requires your body to burn calories. We should all aim to do a combination of aerobic activity and strength exercises each week. There are so many types of exercise – from swimming to dancing, running to walking – and being active in all these different ways has been shown to have countless health benefits, both physical and mental. Exercise is so much more than a weight management tool. It can help you manage stress and enable you to lead a healthy fulfilled life. What's more, it lowers your risk of many diseases, including heart disease, diabetes, obesity, osteoporosis and even some cancers.[28] In fact, people who work out on a regular basis are thought to have up to a 50 per cent lower risk of dying from many of these illnesses.[29]

I always used to find exercise difficult to find time for but I've now made it part of my routine and have seen the positive impact it has on my mood and health. If you find a type of physical activity that you enjoy and that fits easily into your lifestyle, you have a much better chance of keeping it up. Be aware that exercising can stimulate the appetite, meaning that you may end up eating more – or possibly rewarding yourself with treat foods – so just make sure you eat more of the right foods!

THINK FAT LOSS, NOT WEIGHT LOSS

Exercise is often associated with weight loss, but it's fat loss that should be the goal. When you lose weight, you want to maximise fat loss while minimising muscle loss. Know that it is possible to lose body fat without losing much weight on the scales.

If you simply reduce your calorie intake to lose weight, without exercising, you will probably lose muscle as well as fat. When you cut back on calories, your body is forced to find other sources of fuel. In fact, it's been estimated that when people lose weight, about a quarter of the weight they lose is muscle.[30] There are many benefits to following an exercise plan alongside a nutritious diet, as preventing unwanted muscle loss can also help manage the drop in your metabolic rate that happens when you lose weight. It is this rate that often makes it harder to lose weight and keep it off in the long run.

YOU CAN'T OUTRUN A POOR DIET

Eating healthily trumps exercise, pure and simple. Combining exercise with healthy eating is obviously fantastic but problems can occur when you rely on exercise alone. This is partly because of the effect exercise has on our appetite hormones, which make you feel noticeably hungrier after exercise (see page 66).

Planning what you hope to accomplish in each workout can mean the difference between an effective workout and a half-hearted effort. You will also find it easier and see more results if you combine different types of exercise, plus it's more fun. Working out with a friend is a good idea too. They don't just motivate you; they make sure you get to the gym in the first place. It's one thing to cancel plans yourself but it's another to cancel on your friend – they're counting on you!

Working out every day is excessive so you need a routine that allows for rest days (essential for body toning, muscle repair and improving muscle definition) and is manageable in terms of work and social events. Be sensible with your goals. Attempting a 15 mile run in your first week is not a good idea, but alternating between 20 minutes of moderate-intensity exercise such as riding a bike and 30 minutes of low-intensity exercise like walking or swimming is much more likely to be effective. As soon as you feel disciplined enough to diarise your workouts, throw yourself into those HIIT and spinning classes!

ARE YOU OVER EXERCISING?

More often than not, clients who come to my clinic are embarking upon strenuous workouts seven days a week, driven by the goal of shifting unwanted body fat or simply because they are comparing themselves to others. What I tell them is that for most people excessive exercise is unsustainable in the long term and may lead to stress. Adults should aim for 150 minutes of exercise each week. However, there can come a point where exerting more effort actually becomes counter-productive – particularly when it comes to weightlifting. Most people are aware of this concept, but they aren't aware of how to spot it.

TELLTALE SIGNS OF OVER EXERCISING

You're restless at night
If you do a lot of aerobic exercise and are over trained, your sympathetic nervous system can remain excited at all times. This will lead to restlessness and, with an inability to focus, your sleep will be disturbed.

You feel overly sluggish

When you're over trained, your parasympathetic nervous system becomes overly stimulated. This leads to an increase in your stress hormone called cortisol, which leads to both mental and physical fatigue as well as a stubborn tendency to hang on to body fat.

Your muscles always ache

If you are not resting and giving your body a chance to repair your body may be sore and unable to repair itself.

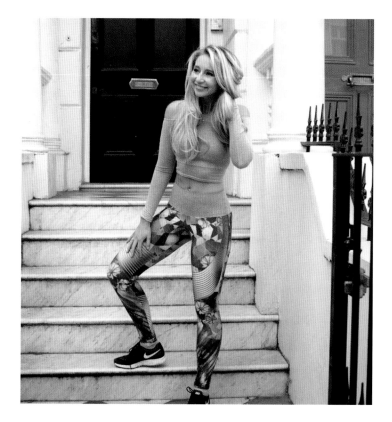

FUELLING FITNESS

Fuelling your body with the right nutrients prior to exercise will give you the energy and strength you need to perform better. Good nutrition will also help your body recover faster after each workout. Refer to A Balanced Plate on pages 56–8 to ensure you are building the right meals. However, it's also important to know when to eat certain foods.

PRE-WORKOUT

Pre-workout meals can be consumed 2–3 hours and up to 30 minutes before workouts. However, choose foods that are easy to digest. Carbs help maximise glycogen stores for high-intensity exercise, while fat helps fuel your body for longer, less intense workouts. Protein may also be included as it improves muscle protein synthesis and helps with recovery. For example, eat an egg on toast with some avocado 2–3 hours before exercising; some Greek yoghurt with fruit is better if you have less than an hour.

POST WORKOUT

After your workout, your body tries to rebuild its glycogen stores and repair torn muscle tissue. Eating the right nutrients soon after you exercise can help your body get this done faster.

When you're working out, your muscles will use up their glycogen stores for fuel so it is important to eat come carbohydrate after your workout, especially if you participate in endurance sports as they cause your body to use more glycogen than resistance training. It is for this reason that runners and swimmers often need to consume more carbs than a weightlifter. You will start to feel lower in energy and your output diminishes as you run low on glycogen stores.

Consuming an adequate amount of protein after a workout gives your body the amino acids it needs to repair and build new muscle tissue.[31] As a rough guide, try to consume up to 0.5 grams per kilogram of protein within 30 minutes of any workout for optimal recovery.[32]

I would suggest eating your main meal if possible within an hour post workout, and if that is not possible try to be prepared and have a source of protein within 30 minutes post workout; think protein shake or some hard-boiled eggs.

WATER

We all know we need to stay hydrated, and especially when exercising. Good hydration has been shown to sustain and even enhance performance, while dehydration has been linked to significant decreases in performance.

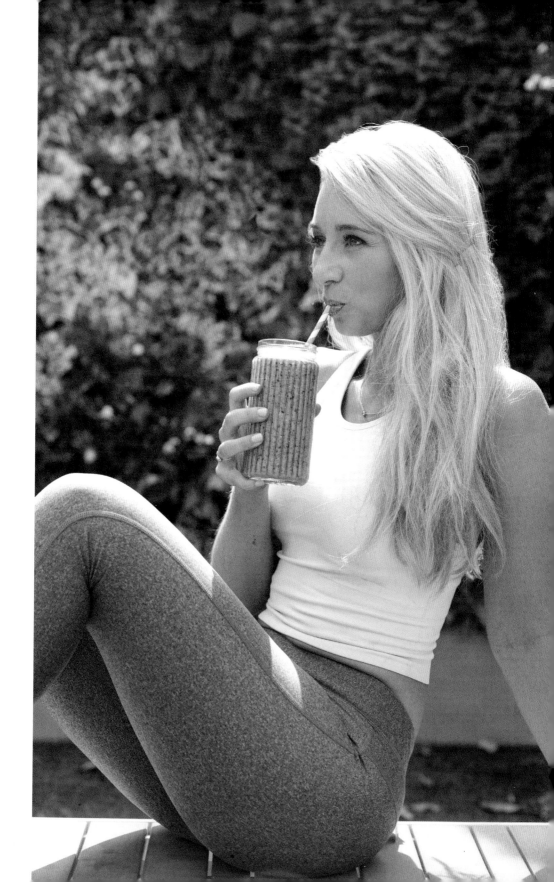

FOOD CLINIC

When a new client books into my clinic, the first thing I do is ascertain whether I am the right person to help them by asking them exactly what their goals are. Detailed questionnaires and a food diary help me build up a picture of each individual's health and medical history, as well as their aims and lifestyle. These take into account general lifestyle, family medical history, digestive health, occupation, immunity, gender specific symptoms and, of course, any medical conditions.

Changing any dietary habits starts with an understanding of why any symptoms have arisen in the first place. Having a complete understanding of someone's health will ensure that nutritional advice is tailored to each person. Ultimately, any nutritional programme should be bespoke, with no 'one plan fits all'.

I think part of my success with clients is my belief in the power of positive nutrition and my reluctance to resort to any scare tactics. I believe in addressing someone's perhaps unrealistic wishes and telling them that what they are practising isn't doing them any favours. For me, it's about finding a practical solution that works for the individual, while being honest and realistic.

Sometimes, a successful consultation can be as simple as hearing that what you're doing now is working for you and all you require are a few small tweaks to your diet to get you to your optimum level. Balance is important in all aspects of life, and too much of anything, even a good thing, can be unhelpful.

UNDERSTANDING YOUR RELATIONSHIP WITH FOOD

There's a very fine line between thinking carefully about what we put into our bodies and obsessing over it and restricting it to dangerous levels. How to regain a healthy relationship with food is a challenge, and the issues surrounding disordered eating deserve a book of their own (see pages 78–9 for more on eating disorders). However, whether your issue is emotional eating, binge eating or you just can't seem to get a handle on the whole nutrition thing, simply learning to identify the underlying problem will help you devise some practical ways to tackle it.

DO YOU COMFORT EAT?

Comfort eating is often used to explain either eating when we're not hungry or overeating. The food may provide a temporary distraction from something painful to us. This can then momentarily change our mood at that time but the relationship between food and mood goes far beyond this specific moment.

I regard emotional eating as a way of dealing with a lack of coping skills. If you are able to spend some time developing new coping strategies, it may help get to the core issue of what is really going on – the emotional issues – and help prevent emotional eating. For many of us, feeling stressed, bored, anxious or sleep-deprived can make us eat (or not eat). This can often then lead to further guilt associated with these behaviours – but we can beat the cycle.

IDENTIFY YOUR TRIGGERS

I often work through the following points with my clients to help them identify their triggers and emotional eating behaviour. Give it a go yourself.

1. Understand your feelings
   What is your eating style? Are there a lot of rules, feelings of guilt or sadness? Did you break one of those dietary rules of yours? If so, have a think about the emotions afterwards and the response. For example, I will not snack between meals; but you were so hungry you couldn't resist that slice of cake in the office. Did you then feel guilty for breaking your rule? Did something stressful happen to you that threw you off your routine?

2. Triggers

We all experience emotions; they help us create behaviours that are necessary for our physical and psychological wellbeing. Everyone is to some degree an emotional eater. The problem occurs when our emotions rule how we eat. See if you can identify yourself in any of the common emotional eating triggers below and then think how these emotional states might affect you throughout your day:

◊ Anger
◊ Anxiety
◊ Worry
◊ Fear
◊ Depression
◊ Negativity
◊ Boredom
◊ Guilt
◊ Shame

3. Challenge any negative thoughts

Many of my clients consider naming that person inside their head that talks to them on a daily basis. You may notice that you bully yourself every day over every decision you make. The sooner you can combat that second voice, the one that tears you down, the better.

4. Reassure yourself with positivity

On the following page is an example of how to turn a diary into positive energy to get you through your day. Keeping a food/mood diary is an excellent way to monitor whether you are actually hungry or whether there is something else at play. You can hopefully see how your environment and events throughout the day can affect your mood and consequently your food choices.

Make a note of the episodes that you consider to be emotional eating. Take a look at the day as a whole and assess it – can you identify a trigger or a general habit? For example, your boss made you stay late at work for an hour and you ate two chocolate bars at your desk even though you were not hungry and had dinner waiting for you at home. Identifying exactly when you are hungry and when you are full can be quite liberating – have you ever really acknowledged this before?

TIME OF DAY	HOW HUNGRY	FOOD/ DRINK	HOW SATISFIED	ANXIETY	LOCATION	COMMENTS
8am	8/10	Porridge and juice	10/10	2/10	At home	Feel okay but guilty as my bowl was very big – then remembered to respect my body's needs.
11am	8/10	Coffee	2/10	8/10	At work	So hungry but want to wait until lunch. Went for a coffee but felt worse; must remember I am allowed to snack when I am hungry.
1pm	10/10	Burger and chips	6/10	10/10	With work colleagues	Very angry for eating a burger – I should have had a mid-morning snack. Must remember it's a learning experience and better to now go for a walk rather than sit here feeling guilty.
4pm	4/10	Hummus and crudites	10/10	3/10	At work	Wasn't hungry but so happy I had my snack, I realised I needed the energy. I feel better but still guilty about lunch.
7pm	6/10	Chicken stir fry with rice	10/10	3/10	At home	Feel proud of myself having a healthy dinner. I'm normally starving when I get home but having the snack helped, I feel like I am listening to my body.
10:30pm	5/10	Ice cream	5/10	10/10	At home	So angry, I craved sugar after an argument with my partner and ate a mini tub of ice cream. I am going to go straight to bed.

LET IT GO

If you didn't eat well today, that's fine, because perfect doesn't exist. It's easy to get upset when something doesn't go the way we hope – it's all too easy to grab something unnecessary to snack on while on the go. Despite knowing that guilt isn't going to help our mindset, we still do it. Often conditioned behaviours are at play so I highly recommend investigating self-love, creating your own luck and living your dreams. If you dream it and then start to believe it, amazing things can happen. We can manifest the thoughts and beliefs and then channel them without even realising it. If we are always telling ourselves 'I won't get that job' or 'I am too fat', then we manifest stress; instead we need to channel the positives – 'I can' and 'I will' – rather than the negatives.

Start every day by being thankful for things you take for granted. Write them down in your own personal journal or make a note on your phone. The list can be as long or as short as you like. Think about how you feel when you're under the weather and you suddenly really appreciate those days when you have your full health. But I think these points are something we can all be grateful for:

◊ The willingness of my mind to learn
◊ My empathy for others
◊ My ability to feel sad and happy
◊ I don't have to go hungry
◊ The setbacks that have formed me and made me stronger

THE BLOOD SUGAR ROLLER COASTER

Any time you eat a carbohydrate, your body digests it, converts it into glucose and sends this glucose into your blood. Glucose is what sugar is called once it is in your blood. If you have ever heard the term 'blood glucose levels', this is the technical term for blood sugar levels. The difference between sugar, refined carbohydrates and whole grains is how long this conversion takes. Foods with lots of fibre (whole grains and fruit) take longer; foods with less or no fibre (white carbs and sugar) digest much more quickly.

When you eat a meal with lots of refined carbohydrates, your pancreas sees a huge spike in blood glucose levels, so it starts to release insulin as quickly as it can to try to catch up. But this can often result in too much glucose being removed from your blood, causing a blood sugar crash, or very low blood sugar levels, which is when you often may want to reach for that biscuit to give you more sugar. For example, having a slice of white bread with jam for breakfast will rarely keep you full for long owing to the rapid release of energy.

When blood sugar levels rise, a person is likely to feel energised at first, but when the sugar levels fall, headaches and nausea may set in, and they can also feel fatigued, irritable, depressed, anxious and nervous.

This is something our bodies do all day, every day – glucose up, glucose down. Our brains depend on it but if we have too much glucose at any one time, from an over-consumption of sugar or carbohydrates (see page 53), insulin may not be able to move it all effectively into cells and our liver has to improvise and do something with it, even if that means storing it on our hips or as cholesterol.

When we overeat or binge eat, it tends to be items that are very high in energy and glucose, I am sure you would all hold your hands up and agree you're more likely to eat too much chocolate than too much broccoli. I find that often the first step to feeling better and towards preventing overeating is to get you off the rollercoaster. So while a sugar rush sounds fun, I encourage you to think twice because what goes in must get processed one way or another.

Blood sugar levels are determined by the type of carbohydrate we eat and what we eat it with. Eating the wrong type of carbohydrate will send you for a ride on the rollercoaster that will leave you feeling low in energy and craving more energy-dense food. Eating the right type of carb will keep you safely off the rollercoaster, allowing you to have happy, energetic and fun moods.

THE EFFECTS OF SUGARY FOODS ON BLOOD SUGAR LEVELS

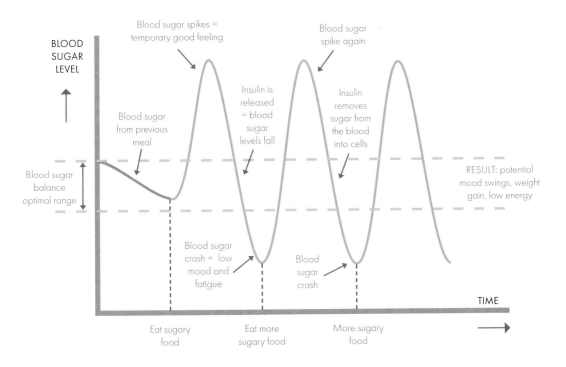

MY TOP 5 TIPS TO BALANCE BLOOD SUGAR LEVELS

◊ Avoid food that is full of refined sugar and switch refined carbs to complex carbs (see Eating the Right Carbs, page 28).

◊ Work on your reliance on stimulants such as caffeine as these may cause a rise in blood sugar.

◊ Start your day well. Aim for a balanced whole grain and protein-rich breakfast with slow-releasing energy (see my porridge recipes on page 120–1).

◊ Enjoy fibre-rich foods at each meal (see page 44).

◊ Consume a varied, nutrient-rich diet to stay happy and healthy throughout the day.

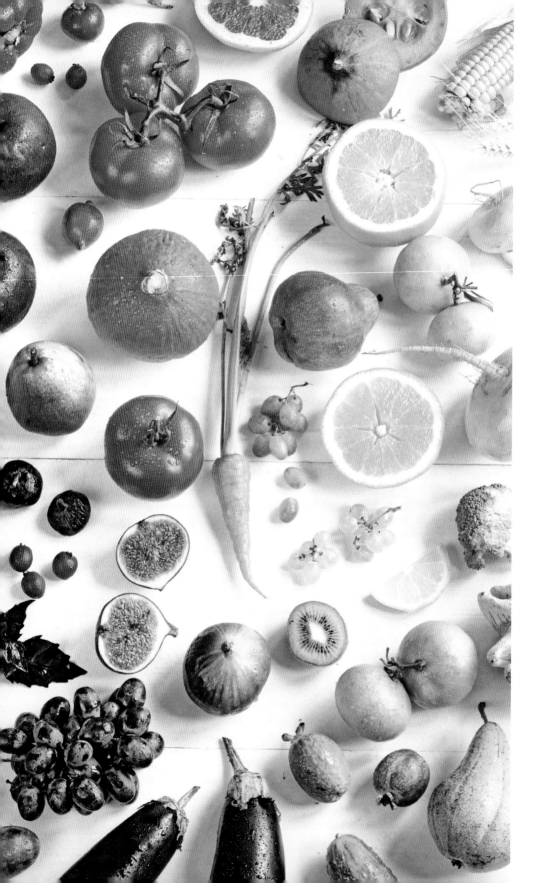

FOOD AND MOOD

Eating a healthy diet can do a lot to improve your mood and sense of wellbeing. In fact, exploring the relationship between what you eat and how you feel can be really effective. Improving your diet can help towards more positive feelings, clearer thinking, more energy and calmer moods. Serotonin is a neurotransmitter in the brain that helps to relay messages from one area of the brain to another. It's believed to influence a variety of psychological and other bodily functions. Most of our brain cells are influenced either directly or indirectly by serotonin. It's also known as our happy hormone and those of us with low serotonin levels are said to feel better when eating sugar. This is obviously not the optimal healthy pathway to alleviate our mood and it often leads to binge eating, not to mention an unhealthy body. Instead you can help serotonin production yourself by consuming plenty of carbohydrate and quality protein containing the amino acid tryptophan.

WHAT IN MY FOOD AFFECTS MY MOOD?

B vitamins

We need B vitamins to get or make energy from our food, otherwise we may feel lethargic and even depressed. B vitamin-rich foods include whole grains, fish and seafood, meat, eggs, milk, leafy green vegetables, beans and peas.

Glucose

The glucose in our blood comes from all the carbohydrates we eat – foods including fruit, vegetables, potatoes, cereals, bread, rice, sugars and lactose in milk.

Omega-3 fatty acids

Good sources of omega-3 are oily fish (salmon, mackerel and sardines), omega-3 eggs (check the box), walnuts and flaxseeds (see pages 35–6 for more on healthy fats).

Tryptophan

An amino acid needed to help make serotonin, which is essential for regulating mood, emotion, sleep and appetite. Find it in bananas, walnuts, turkey, milk, eggs, cheese, brown rice, chicken and fish.

Water

Dehydration can cause headaches, mood changes, fatigue, poor concentration and slower responses.

EATING DISORDERS

Eating disorders are complex mental illnesses with no single cause; they can affect both men and women. Ultimately, many sufferers will require treatment from a number of professionals before being in a position to manage any condition safely.

With all eating disorders, assessing whether a person is being deprived of key nutrients is vital as this can lead to malnutrition, anaemia or an abnormally slow heart rate. Additional health consequences include digestion and fertility issues, hormonal imbalances and impaired bone health. Rigid or restrictive eating patterns will also make it challenging to take part in social activities revolving around food, such as dinner parties or eating out.

Embarking on any diet can mean you are more vulnerable to an eating disorder or will potentially change your relationship with food. It can provide a powerful urge to eat little to nothing or, conversely, to consume excessive quantities of food.

While social media can be a positive space for peer support during recovery from eating disorders, when the overarching emphasis is placed on supposedly healthy diets with 'good' and 'bad' foods, it is obviously an example of where this kind of influence can have a negative effect.

The obsession with meals presented as art and so-called 'clean eating' advice from self-appointed diet gurus is having a tremendous effect on people's relationship with food. There is no doubting now that the bombardment of unqualified diet advice and images of fashionable food can have an unhealthy influence on impressionable people or those already struggling with an eating disorder.[1]

Food is a constant source of inspiration, and while it may be a good thing that people are paying more attention to what they eat, the wealth of information available can be confusing. In my experience, advice from unqualified people has led far too many people to self-diagnose intolerances, often incorrectly.

More and more people are shunning whole food groups based on advice they have read online. Increasingly, I see how some food fads and theories are used as a way of justifying a particular diet and eating disorder.

ORTHOREXIA

Orthorexia is a term first coined as recently as 1996. While it is not currently recognised as a clinical diagnosis, it is a term that can be used to suggest that healthy eating may not be as beneficial as you presume.[2]

Categorised by a pathological obsession for biologically 'pure' food, this preoccupation leads to dietary restrictions. It is often a stage linked to anorexia, with those recovering often naturally falling into orthorexia. Orthorexia always involves an intense compulsion to stick to any single way of eating, thinking and behaving around 'pure' food. For example, sufferers may become so fixated over their macros they cut out vegetables such as red peppers and tomatoes, which are relatively high in sugar and carbohydrates. Many are so obsessed with short-term goals that they don't think about the damage a restricted diet will do in the long term.

People with orthorexia typically cut out entire food groups, often in the mistaken belief they are unhealthy, their bodies are intolerant to them or that eliminating them can cure an ailment. This restriction deprives them of essential nutrition and vitamins. Accompanied by excessive exercise, they are left weak with low energy levels and nutritional deficiencies that can lead to depression and anxiety.

Eating healthily and taking regular exercise are the pillars of a healthy lifestyle, but anything can be dangerous if taken to the extreme.

BODY IMAGE TEST

Take this test to see how body confident you are. How we perceive ourselves really can impact our entire life and happiness.

I feel bad about my appearance...

0 = never   **1** = sometimes   **2** = most of the time   **3** = always

◊ At social gatherings where I know few people
◊ When I look at myself in the mirror
◊ When I am with attractive people
◊ When someone looks at an aspect of my appearance that I don't like
◊ When I try on new clothes
◊ When I exercise
◊ After I have eaten a full meal
◊ When I am wearing revealing clothing
◊ When I step onto the scales to weigh myself
◊ When I think someone has rejected me
◊ When I'm in a sexual situation
◊ When I'm in a bad mood
◊ When I think about how I looked when I was younger
◊ When I see myself in a photo or on a video
◊ When I think I've gained weight
◊ When I think about what I wish I looked like
◊ When I recall hurtful things people have said about my appearance
◊ When I am with people who talk about weight or dieting

TOTAL SCORE: ....

If you have scored higher than 21 you may have poor body confidence but please don't worry, you can work on this and things can only get better! This test is just a useful tool to identify how you currently feel about yourself and whether improvement is required.

SELF LOVE TASKS

No one is perfect. I've had my own battles over my appearance but I have found a passion that has helped me overcome them. As a young, impressionable singer I was told (and believed) that I had to be thin to be successful. Even now I get overwhelmed when I think how far I have come on my journey. It is possible for everyone. We are unique and we need to love, respect and accept who we are. Remove unhelpful inspiration and practise saying these words to yourself:

◊ I am worthy and I am good enough
◊ I accept that only I am in control of my life
◊ No one is perfect; I accept who I am
◊ I do not need to judge myself
◊ No one else is to blame for my own problems

ENHANCE YOUR MEALTIMES

Fall back in love with food and think about your mealtime rituals. Do you rush your food because it's not an enjoyable experience to sit and eat it? Create a new routine by following these guidelines:

◊ Switch off all technology and play some calming music.

◊ Light a candle at the table.

◊ Plate up your food so it's presentable, following The Balanced Plate guidelines.

◊ Use mindful eating techniques (see pages 82–6) to gauge the smell, taste and texture of your food.

◊ Eat slowly and be aware of the environment around you. This may be the first time you have stopped all day and you deserve to relax.

◊ Before you eat, ask yourself how hungry you are. And after you have eaten, ask yourself how satisfied you are and what you are really feeling when you finish your plate.

◊ Give yourself permission to eat. Be at peace with your body, knowing you need nourishment.

◊ Do not compare yourself to others and what they choose to eat.

◊ Try breathing techniques before and after you eat. This may release any guilt surrounding food. Many clients find it effective to say out loud: 'I release this feeling, I let it go.'

MINDFUL EATING

Whenever we eat or drink we have the opportunity to turn our attention to the vivid clarity of this very moment of experience – if we take time to just eat. Too often we feel that eating is something to get over quickly while we multitask. We eat while talking on the phone or working on the computer. We need the simplicity of 'just' eating.

In mindful eating[3], we deliberately direct our full awareness to the bodily sensations, thoughts and emotions that arise and disappear as we eat. Most importantly, we do this without criticism or judgement. We bring clear attention and curiosity to the colours and shapes of our food (as if appreciating a work of art), to the changing fragrances and flavours, to the textures and even the sounds of our food.

A big movement towards mindful eating has begun, suggesting slower and more thoughtful eating can help with weight problems and poor food choices. This is based on the Buddhist approach to mindfulness, which involves being fully aware of what is happening within and around you in the present moment. These techniques have even been used elsewhere to help relieve stress and alleviate problems like high blood pressure and chronic gastrointestinal difficulties. I think it's a fabulous concept and one that we can use to our advantage every day.

Ask yourself how often you engage in the following mindless eating habits:

◊ Using technology at mealtimes
◊ No portion control
◊ Eating food from packets
◊ Eating on-the-go
◊ Not chewing food
◊ Rushing meals
◊ Skipping breakfast
◊ Nighttime munching
◊ Eating on the sofa, instead of at the table
◊ Picking on food throughout the day
◊ Being a moody eater (when angry, bored, tired or stressed)
◊ Being a weekend eater (you're good all week and then at the weekend it goes out the window)
◊ Eating whatever is in the office that day at your desk
◊ Eating heavily processed food

The list goes on and, of course, not everyone is able to avoid these habits all the time, but it's important to be conscious of what you eat, when you eat and how often. Ask yourself whether you feel in control of the decisions you make around food every day? For example, when you go to the cinema, are you aware of how much popcorn you are eating or are you so distracted by the film that you just finish off the whole bucket?

Acknowledging the problem is half the battle. We now need to move forwards and rebuild our relationship with food. I view food as something magical, something to be enjoyed. You are allowed to enjoy your food; we have taste buds for a reason. I say this to a lot of clients who struggle with the term 'earned' food; feeling full is also a natural sensation and doesn't always mean you are bloated, for instance.

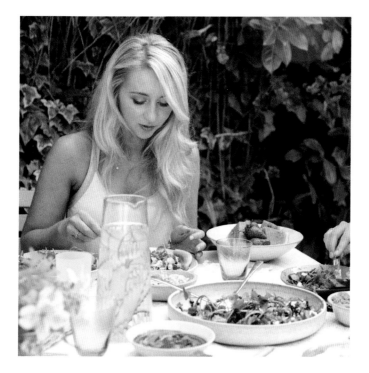

TEST YOURSELF WITH TASTE

Take a piece of fruit, give it a wash and dry it. Before you take your first bite just stop for a second. Ask yourself, out loud if you can: 'Will I enjoy eating this or am I thinking about other things when eating it?'

Now, take that piece of fruit again, sit down and breathe, take in the moment and give it a good once over. What colour is it? What texture? Is it a sweet fruit? What does it make you feel? What does it smell like? There really is so much more to that one piece of food than a quick on-the-go snack.

Next, take a bite of the fruit and chew it for at least 30 seconds (it may feel like an eternity but you should count to 30). Be aware of your breathing to enable you to focus on the fruit entirely. Can you taste it? What is it like to chew and then swallow it? Your usual thoughts as you eat are often what needs to be done that day, where you are off to or what's on the TV in front of you, but this time, it is just you and your fruit.

Just getting into the habit of testing yourself with the taste challenge is a good way to reconnect with food and bring yourself back from the mindless eating which often gets us in trouble and leaves us not feeling our best.

MY TOP 10 TIPS FOR MINDFUL EATING

There are plenty of ways to work mindfulness into your daily food habits. I am a firm believer that finding ways to slow down and eat intentionally are all a part of developing a truly healthy food culture. Mindful eaters tend to have lower body weights, a greater sense of wellbeing and fewer symptoms of eating disorders than those who don't practise mindful eating. But it will only work for you if can make it compatible with your lifestyle. Here are some of my favourite tips to introduce mindfulness to mealtimes in an easy, accessible way. You don't have to do everything at once, take one or two and start implementing them into daily life.

1. Savour the silence
    Take just a few silent moments to call to mind all the people (from farmers to supermarket checkout staff) whose energy has contributed to the food you are about to eat. Visualise them all gathered at your table and thank them. Complete silence may be impossible for a family with children, but you might still encourage some quiet time and reflection. If the family mealtime is too important an opportunity for conversation to pass up, then consider introducing a quiet meal or snack time into your day when you can enjoy it alone. This will give you the best possible start to eating mindfully and encourage you to eat appropriate amounts.

2. Get to know your food

Mindfulness is really about rekindling a relationship with food. From planting a vegetable in the garden to baking homemade bread or visiting a market, it's important to connect with the story behind your food. Even when you have no idea where the food you are eating has come from, try asking yourself some questions about the possibilities. Who grew this? How? Where did it come from? How did it get here? Chances are, you'll not only gain a deeper appreciation for your food, but you'll find your shopping habits changing in the process too.

3. Check you're really hungry

When you feel hungry, just take a second before getting something to eat. Ask yourself this question: 'Am I hungry?' Really think about it and if you're unsure, try waiting 20 minutes. Then ask yourself again to see if you're really and truly hungry. If you feel a snack is needed to keep you going until the next mealtime, think about when you last ate something. If it was less than a few hours ago, it might not really be hunger. Maybe you just need a break to stretch your legs or a drink of water instead.

4. Be kind to your stomach

Too often we live at a distance from our bodies. Before you take your first servings of food, bring your attention to your stomach. Ask yourself how much would it be comfortable working with? Try serving yourself two-thirds of any typical amount to begin with. After you've eaten it, check in with your stomach again. How full is it? While your tongue may say it wants more to taste, does the stomach really want more to work with?

5. Pay attention

Paying attention to the details of our food can be a great way to start eating mindfully. Savour the first few bites of food or sips of liquid. When you eat on the go or wolf down your meals, it can be hard to notice what you are even eating, let alone truly savour all the different sensations of eating it. Whatever you're eating, consciously engage with the texture of it in your mouth, the smells, colour and temperature. If you are trying to introduce mindful eating to your family, consider talking more about the flavours and textures of food. Ask yourself what the tastes are like and share your observations and opinions too.

6. Slow down

It's a good idea to remind yourself, and your family, that eating is not a race. Taking the time to savour and enjoy your food is one of the healthiest things you can do. You are more likely to notice when you are full, you'll chew your food more and hence digest it more easily and you'll probably find yourself noticing flavours you might otherwise have missed. A fun way to slow down is to try eating with your non-dominant hand or try putting down your knife and fork between bites.

7. Give your food your full attention

    Our daily lives are full of distractions, and it's not uncommon for us to eat with the TV blaring
    or have someone fiddling with their phone. Consider making mealtimes family time by eating
    together and in an electronics-free zone. I'm not saying you should never eat pizza in front of the
    TV, but that too should be a conscious choice that marks the exception, not the norm. I challenge
    you to try it and give your meal your undivided attention.

8. Limit temptation

    Pre-portion your food so you're not tempted to eat more than you need to. When you're busy and
    you need to eat on-the-go, it can be tempting to skip a meal or grab a convenient snack. But rather
    than let those moments catch you out, have foods to hand that are healthy and pre-portioned.
    That way you're not going to accidentally eat too much without realising it. Also consider keeping
    certain problematic foods out of the house, where they will just ask to be eaten.

9. Are you full yet?

    Being mindful when eating focusses your attention so you can register when you've eaten
    enough and are satisfied. Slowing down and learning to recognise when you're full can help
    stop weight gain, indigestion and any bloated, sluggish feelings.

10. Make the time

    My final point is really important. I urge you to make time for your meals as they are essential
    to your health and wellbeing. I know what it's like to be busy, but making time for regular meals
    will keep you energised throughout your day, fuelling your body and mind. Mindful eating does
    not have to be an exercise in super-human concentration, but rather a simple commitment to
    appreciating, respecting and, above all, enjoying the food you eat. Introduce it at home, at work,
    or even as you snack while out and about. When the focus becomes how you eat, not what you
    eat, you may find your notions of what you want to eat shifting dramatically for the better too.

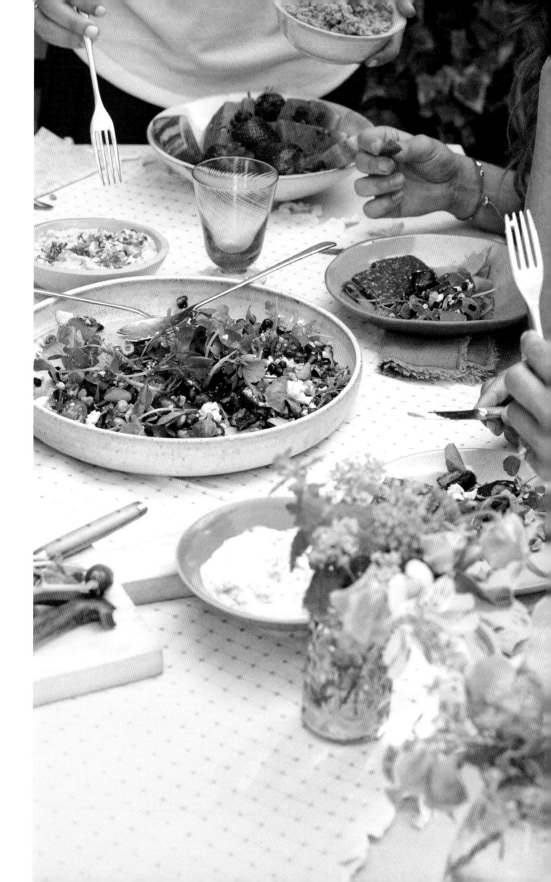

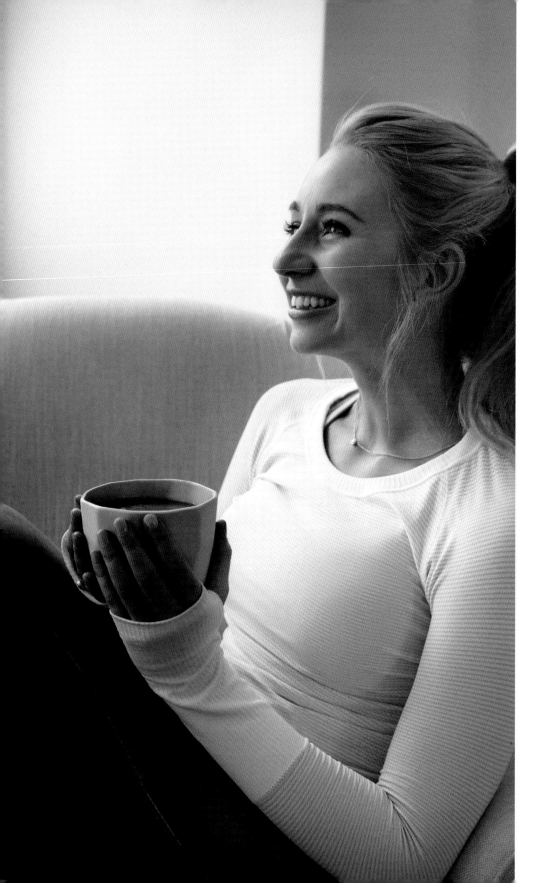

SLEEP

Never underestimate the power of sleep. We all love it but rarely do we get enough each night. The alarm goes off, we hit snooze and we feel like we haven't woken up all day. The irony is that all too many people forego sleep in the name of productivity. Sleep deprivation hurts you both physically and emotionally, yet the myth exists that we can do our jobs just as well on four, five or six hours of sleep as we can on seven or eight, which is simply not true.

Every night, I set aside some time to wind down into my routine. First, I'll turn off my phone 30 minutes before bedtime and leave it outside the bedroom. I often take a hot bath as it seems to slow down my brain and winds down my body. A warm drink really helps me to relax too. I always get into dedicated pyjamas instead of old bed-gym clothes. I also talk to my partner about a few things I'm thankful for that day, giving the day a closing scene. Ending the day with positive thinking makes for better sleep.

THE IMPORTANCE OF SLEEP

One of the first things I ask my clients is how much sleep they get. We may need to work on important dietary aspects, but sleep can affect so much more than energy levels.

Repair and replenish
Sleep is important for various aspects of brain function. This includes cognition, concentration, productivity and performance. All of these are negatively affected by sleep deprivation. Good sleep, on the other hand, has been shown to improve problem-solving skills and enhance memory performance of both children and adults.

Weight
People with short sleep duration tend to weigh significantly more than those who get adequate sleep. The effect of sleep on weight gain is believed to be mediated by numerous factors, including hormones and motivation to exercise. Studies show that sleep-deprived individuals have a bigger appetite and tend to eat more calories.

Mood
Those who suffer from depression often complain about sleep quality. Without sleep, your mood is without doubt impacted negatively.

MY SUCCESSFUL SLEEP TIPS

Routine

Your body has a natural time-keeping clock known as your circadian rhythm, which functions on a set loop, aligning itself with sunrise and sunset. It affects your brain, body and hormones, helping you stay awake and telling your body when it's time to sleep. Being consistent with your sleep and waking times can aid in sleep quality in the long term. If you struggle with sleep, try to get in a habit of waking up and going to bed at a similar time each day and night. After several weeks, you may not even need an alarm. Natural sunlight or bright light during the day helps keep your circadian rhythm healthy. This improves daytime energy, as well as nighttime sleep quality and duration.

Technology detox

Artificial lighting and electronics emit light of a blue wavelength, which tricks our brains into thinking it's daytime. A part of the brain called the pineal gland secretes the hormone melatonin, which signals to our bodies and brains that it is time to go to sleep. Blue light is very effective at inhibiting melatonin production, reducing both the quantity and quality of our sleep. Your phone may well be the hardest habit of them all to curb but it will be the most effective; try putting it as far away from your bed as possible and then work up to switching it off an hour before bed. One good tip is to buy an alarm clock so you are not using your phone.

Environment

I believe that your environment can really help if you want to get a good night's sleep. This can include aspects such as temperature, noise, furniture choice and arrangement, external lights and more. To optimise your bedroom environment, try to minimise external noise, light and artificial lights from devices like alarm clocks. Make sure your bedroom is a quiet, clean, relaxing and enjoyable place.

Exercise

Exercise is wonderful for the body and can help us with our sleep – unless you are doing it just before bedtime as the induced alertness and hormones like epinephrine or adrenaline can keep you awake. My advice is to exercise no later than 3 hours before bedtime.

Food

Late-night eating may negatively impact both sleep quality and the natural release of growth hormones and melatonin. However, a high-carb meal eaten a few hours before bedtime may help you fall asleep faster and improve sleep quality. This is likely due to its effect on the hormone tryptophan, which can make you feel tired. Ultimately, you are unique and you need to find what works for you.

Diary

If you can't slow your mind and meditation isn't your thing, try removing the thoughts from your head and putting them on paper.

Coffee

Caffeine does have its benefits but consuming it up to six hours before bed can significantly worsen sleep quality.[4]

Yoga or meditation

Relaxation techniques before bed have been shown to improve sleep quality and are another common technique used to treat insomnia. Try stretching in your pyjamas before bed and engaging in some deep breathing with a scented candle lit.

Hot drinks

We are all different – some find it best to avoid liquids before bed but I personally find a hot cacao drink or a calming chamomile herbal tea can really help. Lots of herbal remedies are said to induce sleep, so find one that you like and give it a go.

Bath

This has to be my favourite, especially if you add Epsom salts to the water – the magnesium helps soothe sore muscles. A hot bath 90 minutes before bed can significantly improve sleep quality.[5] If you're not a bath person, a hot shower can have a similar effect.

Avoid alcohol and sugar

Drinking alcohol at night can really affect your sleep and hormones. Alcohol is known to cause or increase the symptoms of sleep apnea, snoring and disrupted sleep patterns. It also alters nighttime melatonin production. Sugar highs are not going to help either. Make smart choices in the evenings particularly, if you are eating later than usual.

RE-NOURISH
MENU

Now that you've identified and learnt more about your relationship with food, it's time to re-nourish. I am going to take you through this journey and leave you with an example of how to enjoy a healthy balanced week of food. We will be stocking your cupboards with the right items, discussing your goals and introducing healthy hacks to keep you motivated and make eating well as simple as possible.

Remember this is about learning to cook and enjoy simple, delicious food; this is not a diet plan. Forget everything you have tried before and let me get you back to basics. A life full of energy, happiness and satisfaction awaits you when you re-nourish your mind and body.

CONSISTENCY IS CRUCIAL

For any healthy regime to be a success, you must be consistent over a prolonged period of time. It's worth tracking your progress using measurements of key body parts rather than weight. Even if you are becoming slimmer and more toned, the numbers on the scales may still increase (or stay as they are) due to increased muscle mass. Don't be disheartened; your body composition will be changing. You should simply judge your body improvements by how comfortable you feel in your clothes. While it may take weeks before friends or family notice a difference, you will be aware of changes more quickly.

You don't become overweight by eating the occasional chocolate bar or piece of cake if you have an otherwise good diet. Both putting on weight and slimming down to a healthy weight (and then maintaining it) really come down to a consistent lifestyle. As we have already explored, successfully losing weight is more about changing or adapting unhealthy patterns than measuring the precise calorie content of every food you eat.

It really is very simple: aim to eat a healthy, balanced diet and build some activity into your daily life. Don't skip meals, as you will be tempted to over-compensate later. Instead, eat regular meals, especially breakfast, and make sure your portion sizes are appropriate.

If you are hungry by 11am then have a snack but make sure it is a sensible choice, something to enhance your day. I often advise a protein-based snack or something high in fibre that will help keep you fuller for longer (see pages 204–17 for more snack ideas). If you cut out entire food groups, there can be some seriously negative consequences, such as nutrition deficiencies, which can affect your health. No single food contains all the nutrients you need to stay healthy, so it's important to eat a range of foods every day.

Although some diets have their merits, don't be tempted to make drastic changes overnight. If you try to change all your habits immediately, it may be too much too soon. Focus on a few small changes, step by step, which is likely to be more effective in the long term. For example, if you're used to always having a dessert after dinner, swap your usual creamy or sweet pudding for fruit (although the occasional dessert is definitely allowed!). Make small changes and you will eventually be rid of all the bad habits that may have crept into your life. You will then be free to make some real and lasting changes, such as adopting mindful eating habits.

BE PREPARED

We develop habits because they save us time and energy and often because they give us a sense of comfort and reward. But what if you could change your habits so that you could start eating more healthily automatically, without ever having to think about it? You can, and it's easier than you think.

Being too busy is the main reason people give for opting for heavily processed foods and ready meals. So, planning and preparing your meals ahead of time is hugely beneficial to maintaining a healthy lifestyle. If time is short in the morning, choose a quick and easy breakfast such as porridge topped with natural yoghurt – it only takes a few minutes to prepare yet still provides a good intake of healthy carbohydrates and protein. Or maybe make something the night before, like my overnight oats (see page 121.) An easy approach to packing a healthy lunchbox is to make batches of cooked vegetables, grains and meat or fish – freezing them in portions to be defrosted the day before use makes them last longer too (see page 164 for some easy lunchbox ideas).

And think about what you're going to have for dinner in advance – not when you're hungry on the way home after a long day on your feet! Maybe take a portion of fish or meat out of the freezer in the morning, leaving it to defrost by the time you get home after work. Having a plan of what your final meal of the day will consist of will prevent you from shopping badly (or stopping at the local takeaway). Healthy meals really can be just as satisfying as the alternatives (if not more so); it's just about taking the time to prepare them.

RECIPE CLINIC

While complete diet makeovers can be overwhelming, focussing on small, simple changes and swaps makes healthy eating more manageable and sustainable over the long term. Instead of throwing your kitchen, eating habits and sanity upside down, focus on making your mealtimes more nutritious.

Avocado toast

While this is super-tasty it is not providing you with anywhere near enough protein. Avocados contain around 2g of protein per 100g, which is not going to help you reach your requirements for the day.

DIY: Add a poached egg or two, some smoked salmon or, if you are vegetarian or vegan, try it topped with some edamame. These contain around 8g of protein per 100g – with the added bonus of 7g of dietary fibre.

Banana toast

I see a lot of banana toast breakfasts and they do look delicious but they may not keep you full. A breakfast of just a slice of toast and a banana (more often than not with added honey) is going to be lacking in that key macronutrient: protein.

DIY: Simply sprinkle your toast with seeds and crushed nuts, or spread a small amount of nut butter on the toast before placing the banana on top; that way you get a boost of healthy fats and protein.

Porridge

I love a tasty bowl of porridge with fruit and milk but again this is lacking in protein and healthy fats, especially if it's eaten plain. Although oats are a good source of protein, it is best to boost the levels further when adding fruit.

DIY: Add some seeds and nuts to your bowl. Seeds can contain up to 19g of protein per 100g and nuts 20g per 100g (depending on the variety of seed and nut, of course). This will also give you a healthy boost of fatty acids. If you have a nut allergy, or it's just not your thing, then add a dollop of Greek yoghurt, which has roughly 10g of protein per 100g, again dependent upon the brand.

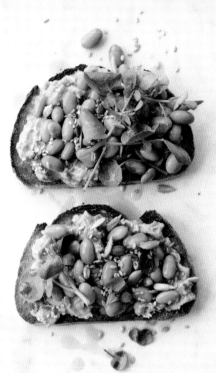

page 128

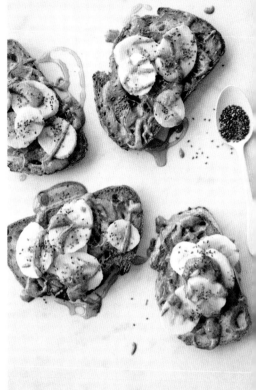

page 131

pages 120–1

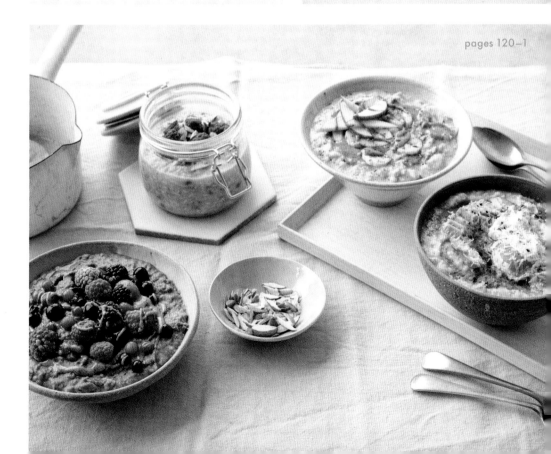

Breakfast smoothie/juice

With lots of fruit and veg and even healthy fats, this can be a fab option but it may not be fulfilling your needs for the day. Gauge how active you are and think about the rest of the day ahead. If you're not blitzing in nuts or avocado then it is unlikely this will be a balanced meal option for you and is better viewed as a side or snack. Be mindful though that you don't find yourself drinking lots of smoothies every day, as that's far too much sugar.

DIY: Always add some carbohydrate, perhaps blend in some oats, and then add a scoop of protein powder to keep you fuller for longer and balance those blood sugar levels!

Courgetti bowls

These taste amazing and are fine for a light meal but are not very nutritionally balanced. They often lack sufficient protein, carbohydrate and fats.

DIY: Ensure you add a generous portion of protein and a drizzle of olive oil if you are missing some healthy fats. I often mix my pasta bowls with half spaghetti and half courgetti to create a base for my veggie chilli (see page 182).

Acai bowl

This is now the trendy healthy go-to when eating out for breakfast. It's starting to catch on at home too, with more shops selling frozen acai blends. The problem is that it's a sugar fest; this bowl is almost like ice cream with tons of fruit and no protein or healthy fats.

DIY: Make sure you only have this bowl occasionally. It is unlikely to keep you full unless you generously apply more toppings such as nuts, nut butter and seeds, or even a scoop of protein powder, for added protein and fats.

Brownies

There isn't really a way around this; brownies contain sugar. Just because they are made with perceived healthier ingredients doesn't make it nutritious.

DIY: My tip is to embrace the treat but try making them with sweet potato for extra fibre and nutrients. You are now choosing it to enjoy your chocolate fix with the added benefits of nourishing your body, not as a food item replacement alone.

SMART SWAPS

Bagel	⟶	Rye bread
Biscuits	⟶	Oatcakes
Breakfast bars	⟶	Homemade breakfast bars
Cereal	⟶	Oats
Chips	⟶	Potato wedges
Crisps	⟶	Veggie crisps
Croissant	⟶	Wholemeal scone
Fruit yoghurt	⟶	Natural yoghurt with berries
Granola	⟶	Muesli (or my Homemade Granola)
Ice cream	⟶	Frozen banana
Latte	⟶	Cappuccino
Lettuce	⟶	Spinach
Margarine	⟶	Butter
Milk chocolate	⟶	Dark chocolate
Pasta	⟶	Wholegrain pasta
Sour cream	⟶	Greek yoghurt
Tomato soup	⟶	Minestrone
White rice	⟶	Quinoa

HEALTHY HACKS

It is important to remember that food is meant to be enjoyed. Eating out, getting a takeaway and hosting a dinner for friends are all social occasions that should be viewed as fun, not something to make you feel guilty. It can be easy to get carried away though, when you are surrounded by other people or when faced with a long menu, leading you to make some unhealthy choices. Although this is, of course, perfectly fine from time to time, if you eat out often or like to host regularly, here are a few tips to keep you on track.

EATING OUT

There is nothing more pleasurable than a meal shared with those closest with you. In fact, most of our celebrations revolve around food. Life and what we eat are to be enjoyed, and eating out is one of my favourite things to do.

These days, there are loads of amazing options on menus to cater for all tastes and preferences. Here are a few tips for making healthier choices – but if you're out for a pizza, then just go ahead and enjoy it!

◊ Include plenty of vegetables or salad in your meal
◊ Avoid adding extra salt
◊ Consider going for grilled or steamed options
◊ Swap chips for new potatoes, extra vegetables or salad
◊ Ask for dressings and sauces to be served on the side
◊ Ask for less oil (they may not be using healthy oils in the kitchen)
◊ Reduce your intake of deep-fried food (e.g. dumplings, prawn toast or battered items)
◊ Limit over-sweetened dishes like sweet and sour dishes
◊ Consider opting for veg-based sauces rather than creamy sauces
◊ Opt for wholegrain over white bread
◊ Limit condiments like ketchup, satay sauce, mayonnaise or BBQ sauce as these contain extra sugars, salts and fats

THE DINNER PARTY

If you're the type of person who lets others make decisions for you, then you may need to give yourself a nudge. I have one client in particular who springs to mind here, who has the warmest soul and would go out of her way to ensure her guests had everything they wanted. She would buy chocolates for dessert, make food she wasn't comfortable eating and put herself through a night of raised tension, anxiety, guilt and then shame. This led to a day of restriction the next day to compensate for the night before. It does not have to be like that; you can make your own decisions. Here's how:

1. Ask your guests to bring their own drinks – soft drinks, wine and beer – so you can stick to your choices.

2. Make lots of healthy side dishes and one big main dish; you can then dish your own portion onto your plate and mix the ratio of food. If you make something like a big pastry pie you can have however much you want with extra vegetables.

3. Always have two desserts; I usually prepare a healthy fruit option (which still tastes fab) and a healthy twist on an indulgent dessert (see pages 190–9). Often no one even bats an eyelid and they tend to go for the fruit too!

4. Create an atmosphere: put the music on, light some candles and remember this is social time. It's not just about the food; take time to enjoy the company you are with.

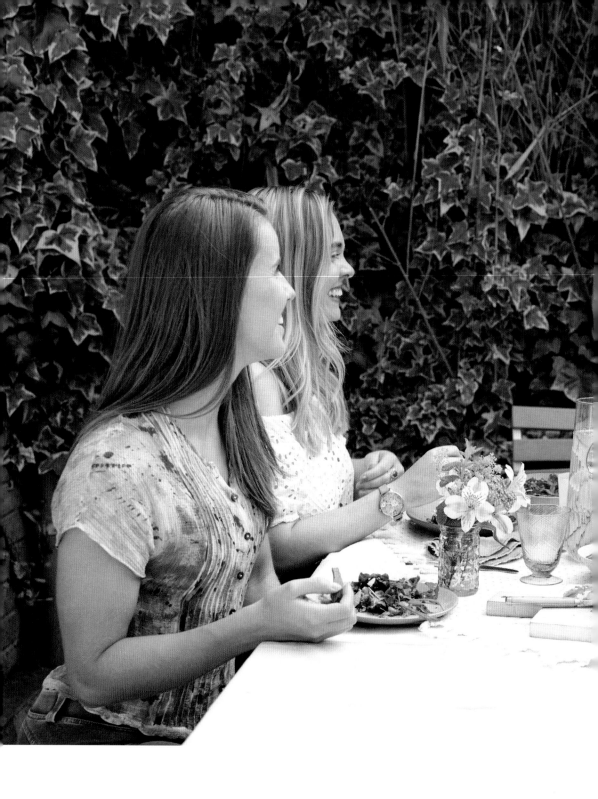

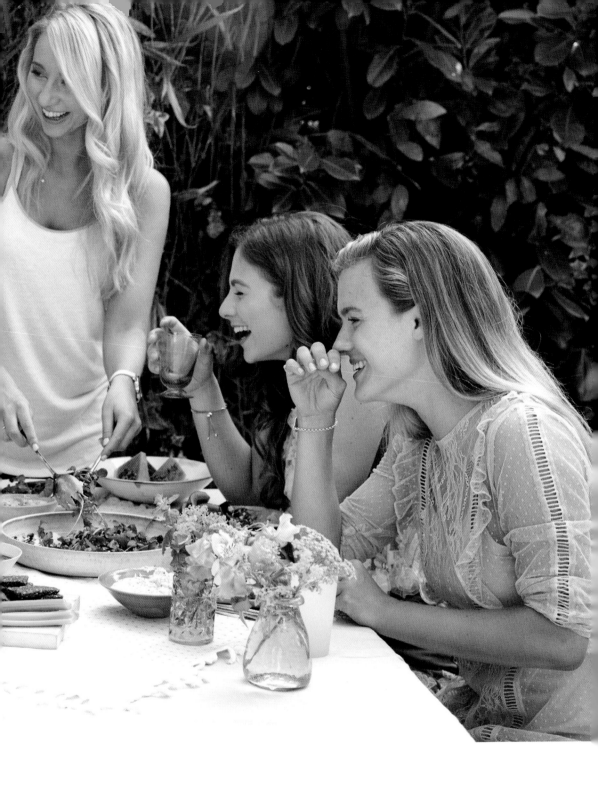

RE-NOURISH GUIDELINES

There are no rules when it comes to re-nourishing. Enjoying what you eat is the only way you'll be able to keep it up. One day at a time, push yourself to live more healthily than the previous day. Think nutrients, not numbers.

KITCHEN DETOX

Before you head to the supermarket for your first healthy shop, make sure you remove your share of unnatural and heavily processed foods from the cupboards. For those of you who have quite a few unhealthy things lurking in the kitchen, it may be best to do this in stages. Perhaps tackle the freezer one week, the cupboards the following week and finally the fridge. If you are concerned about wastage, think about donating items to a food bank, or consider using them up before you embark on your healthy shop.

You're now ready to tackle the supermarket. A good tip to remember is that the natural, healthier products tend to live on the outer edges of the shop with the tempting confectionary aisle usually located in the centre, so in order to resist temptation, try to avoid these aisles altogether.

SHOPPING

Eating more healthily and saving money while doing it may sound too good to be true, but it's really not. Devising a regular shopping list (and planning your meals ahead of time, see page 95) will stop you buying things you don't really need. Before heading out, spend a few minutes looking in your kitchen cupboards and then write a list. Be sure to organise it by category so you're not zigzagging all over the supermarket. Also, have a nutritious snack like some almonds just before heading out – you won't even think twice about lifting anything unnecessary off the shelf.

As you walk through the supermarket aisles, checking items off your shopping list, you may well think that you're picking healthy products for you and the family. Yet, as we become more health-conscious, food manufacturers have found new and creative ways to pass off their not-so-healthy products as nutritious (and, unfortunately, they've become really quite good at it). It's a real challenge to identify a truly healthy food without looking at the label. As a general rule, always check the label and keep to buying fresh produce as much as possible.

HOW TO READ LABELS

Nutrition labels are often displayed as a panel or grid on the back or side of the packaging. For example, the image below shows the nutrition label on a loaf of white bread.

Nutrition				
Typical values	100g contains	Each slice (typically 44g) contains	% RI*	RI* for an average adult
Energy	985kJ	435kJ		8400kJ
	235kcal	105kcal	5%	2000kcal
Fat	1.5g	0.7g	1%	70g
of which saturates	0.3g	0.1g	1%	20g
Carbohydrate	45.5g	20.0g		
of which sugars	3.8g	1.7g	2%	90g
Fibre	2.8g	1.2g		
Protein	7.7g	3.4g		
Salt	1.0g	0.4g	7%	6g

This pack contains 16 servings
*Reference intake of an average
adult (8400kJ/2000kcal)

This type of label includes information on energy (kJ/kcal), fat, saturates (saturated fat), carbohydrate, sugars, protein and salt. It may also provide additional information on certain nutrients, such as fibre. All nutrition information is provided per 100g and sometimes per portion. There are guidelines that will indicate whether a food is high or low in fat, saturated fat, salt or sugar. These are:

Total fat
High: more than 17.5g of fat per 100g
Low: 3g of fat or less per 100g

Saturated fat
High: more than 5g of saturated fat per 100g
Low: 1.5g of saturated fat or less per 100g

Sugars
High: more than 22.5g of total sugars per 100g
Low: 5g of total sugars or less per 100g

Salt
High: more than 1.5g of salt per 100g (or 0.6g sodium)
Low: 0.3g of salt or less per 100g (or 0.1g sodium)[5]

ORGANIC FOOD

The organic food market saw its fifth year of consecutive growth in 2016. A great many people now think organic food is safer, healthier and tastier than regular food. Others say it's better for the environment and improves animal welfare. Is it all marketing hype or is organic food worth the higher price?

The term organic simply refers to the process of how certain foods are produced. Organic agriculture is bound by legal regulations that restrict the use of artificial chemicals, hormones, antibiotics or genetically modified organisms. In addition, all produce is free from artificial food additives, including artificial sweeteners, preservatives, colourings and flavourings.

Ultimately, there is not enough strong evidence available to prove that eating organic provides health benefits over eating regular foods and so whether you choose to buy organic or not is a personal choice.

I choose to eat some organic food but certainly not exclusively, as it's definitely not essential for good health. Having said that, I always try to buy organic, free-range eggs and meats along with sustainably sourced fish.

It's good to remember that a thorough rinsing of any fruit or vegetables with tap water will go a long way towards washing off any pesticide residues. It is also reassuring to know that in the UK we are subject to some of the strictest regulations for pesticides in the world.

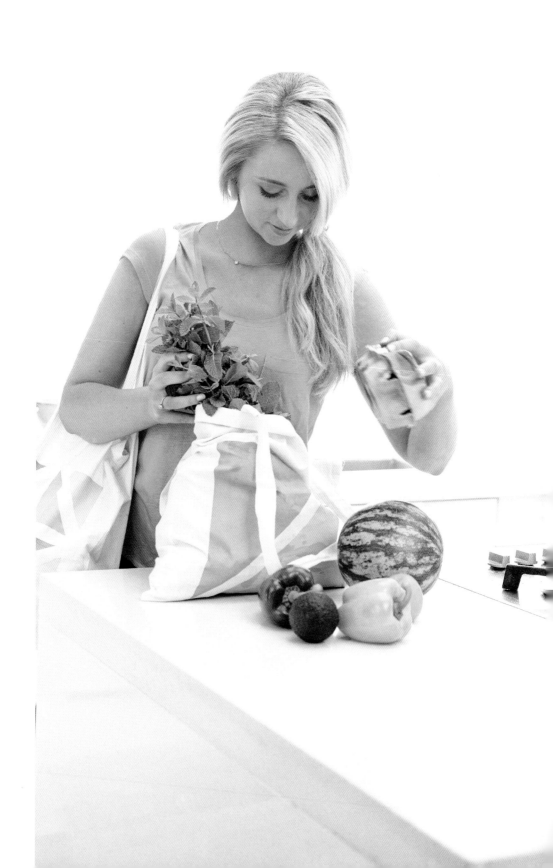

MY FAVOURITE INGREDIENTS

By making a space for each of the main food groups, you'll ensure you get a good variety of nutritious, nourishing ingredients into your diet. Also, by specifically shopping by food groups, you eliminate (or at least reduce) the chance of filling your trolley with heavily processed foods. Here are some of my favourite ingredients that I aim to eat as often as I can or to have in my store cupboard ready to make into a quick dinner.

VEGETABLES	FRUIT	SPICES AND HERBS
Artichoke	Apples	Allspice
Asparagus	Bananas	Basil
Aubergine	Berries	Bay leaves
Avocado	Cherries	Black peppercorns
Broccoli	Figs	Chilli
Brussels sprouts	Grapefruit	Cinnamon
Cabbage	Kiwi fruit	Coriander
Carrot	Lemons	Cumin
Cauliflower	Limes	Curry powder
Celery	Melon	Garlic
Courgettes	Oranges	Ginger
Cucumber	Peaches	Mint
Fennel	Pears	Oregano
Garlic	Plums	Paprika
Green beans	Pomegranate	Parsley
Kale		Rosemary
Leeks		Sea salt
Lettuce		Thyme
Mushrooms		Turmeric
Onion		
Peppers		
Rocket		
Spinach		
Spring onion		
Sweet potato		
Tomatoes		

CONDIMENTS, SPREADS AND OILS	FRIDGE	PROTEIN
Coconut oil	Butter	Beef
Kimchi	Dairy milk	Chicken
Miso paste	Unsweetened fortified plant-based milks (almond/coconut/hemp)	Eggs
Mustard		Fish
Nut butter (see page 243)	White cheese (mozzarella/feta)	Good-quality protein powder
Olive oil	Yoghurt (Greek or natural with no added sugar)	Tinned sardines/mackerel/salmon
Passata		Tofu
Sauerkraut		Tuna
Soy sauce		Turkey
Tahini		
Tamari (gluten free)		
Tomato ketchup (see page 241)		
Vinegar (apple cider, balsamic, red wine and white wine)		

CUPBOARDS	FLOURS	SWEETENERS/ BONUS ITEMS
Brown pasta	Almond	Cacao powder
Brown rice	Coconut	Chia seeds
Buckwheat	Wholemeal	Desiccated coconut
Chickpeas		Flaxseeds
Lentils		Honey
Nuts and seeds		Maple syrup
Oatcakes		Stevia
Oats		Vanilla bean paste
Pearl barley		
Quinoa		
Rice cakes		
Tinned beans		
Vermicelli rice noodles		

SEASONAL EATING

Eating in season it is a great way of ensuring you get a varied diet and of maximising optimum nutrition. Locally sourced seasonal food is often cheaper, as well as being better for the environment since it hasn't had to be transported across the globe. Of course, things that can't be grown in this country need to be imported, but they still have their own local season. Here's a guide to when foods are at their best.

	FRUIT	VEG
SPRING	Apricots, Bananas, Grapefruit, Oranges, Rhubarb	Artichoke, Asparagus, Broad beans, Cabbage, Cauliflower, Chicory, Leeks, Peas, Peppers, Potatoes, Purple sprouting broccoli, Radish, Spinach, Spring onions
SUMMER	Apricots, Bananas, Blueberries, Cherries, Melons, Nectarines, Peaches, Raspberries, Strawberries	Asparagus, Aubergine, Beetroot, Broad beans, Broccoli, Cabbage, Carrots, Celery, Courgettes, Cucumber, Fennel, Garlic, Peas, Peppers, Potatoes, Radish, Runner beans, Spinach, Spring onions, Sweetcorn, Tomatoes
AUTUMN	Apples, Bananas, Blackberries, Blueberries, Clementines, Cranberries, Figs, Grapes, Melons, Pears, Plums	Aubergine, Beetroot, Broccoli, Brussels sprouts, Butternut squash, Cabbage, Carrots, Cavolo nero, Celeriac, Celery, Courgettes, Fennel, Garlic, Kale, Leeks, Onions, Parsnips, Peppers, Potatoes, Pumpkins, Radish, Runner beans, Swede, Sweet potato, Tomatoes
WINTER	Apples, Bananas, Clementines, Cranberries, Forced rhubarb, Grapefruit, Lemons, Oranges, Pears, Pomegranates	Artichoke, Beetroot, Brussels sprouts, Butternut squash, Cabbage, Cauliflower, Celeriac, Celery, Chicory, Kale, Leeks, Onions, Parsnips, Purple sprouting broccoli, Red cabbage, Swede, Sweet potato

FISH	MEAT
Cod, Crab, Haddock, Mackerel, Pollock, Sardines, Scallops, Sea bass, Sea trout, Wild salmon	Beef, Chicken, Lamb
Crab, Haddock, Mackerel, Plaice, Pollock, Sardines, Sea bass, Sea trout, Tuna, Wild salmon	Beef, Chicken
Clams, Crab, Haddock, Halibut, Mussels, Oysters, Pollock, Sardines, Sea bass, Sea trout	Beef, Chicken, Game, Turkey
Haddock, Oysters, Sardines, Scallops, Sea bass, Sea trout	Beef, Chicken, Duck, Goose, Venison

A SAMPLE WEEKLY MENU

I have deliberately designed a menu and not a plan like so many other healthy eating books. I don't believe set plans are realistic, nor do they fulfil or meet everybody's individual needs and preferences. Instead, I've set out a sample menu that follows my balanced plate principles – follow these whenever you can (see page 114 for my sample menu and pages 56–9 for more on A Balanced Plate).

I have designed this menu based on the recipes I've included in this book. Obviously, if you want to have a dessert on a Wednesday instead of a Monday then just swap it around; it is totally interchangeable. And whether you are a vegan, vegetarian or flexitarian, you can easily adjust each meal to suit your needs – or substitute a meal for another from this book. All of the meals have been carefully designed to be well balanced in terms of protein, carbs and fats so you can be sure you're getting optimum benefits from each one and won't be missing out on key nourishment.

I am not the sort who believes in zero sugar forever and always. I honestly love dessert as much as the next person. It's all about moderation and, of course, adaptation. I would never advise having dessert every day (perhaps once or twice a week) but it depends on your lifestyle and goals. If your goal isn't weight loss, then there are lots of healthier desserts that you can enjoy. However, if weight loss is key, then you need to be mindful of your overall energy intake.

If you adjust the portion sizes to fit your needs (using the hand portion diagram on page 57) this menu will leave you feeling energised, satisfied, free from sugar cravings and, after a short period of time, sleeping better too.

By following these guidelines for just seven days you will be amazed that you can eat normal, healthy portions of every food group, you will be in a productive routine, perform optimally at work, sleep better and feel energised. If you are someone who has had a history of bingeing or restricting or following fad diets, this is going to change your life!

I highly recommend following this basic structure for at least seven days, then continue to four weeks if you can, by which stage you will definitely feel re-nourished! It is designed to give you more time for your meals in the evening and at the weekends.

This menu should be prepared for in advance, so make sure you check the day before that you have the correct ingredients in the fridge. If worse comes to the worst, just double up on dinner and take a portion to work the next day.

I highly recommend removing caffeine and alcohol from your diet – or at least reducing it – just for seven days. Be prepared for some withdrawal symptoms if you rely heavily on these. I think there is a place for these items in everyone's diet but it is important to know that you can survive without them and let your body be free from stimulants for a short period of time. This is, of course, optional but I suggest giving it a go to feel more energised throughout the week.

Each meal in this book includes adequate amounts of protein, healthy carbohydrates, colour and a small amount of healthy fat. However, do change the size of the carbohydrate and protein according to your day. For example, if you have been sitting down all day at a desk, you may not need as much rice (carbohydrate) at dinner; extra veg will be enough. Check the diagram of portion sizes on page 57. I often recommend reducing the starchy/complex carbohydrates by half (particularly if you haven't been very active) and if that still feels like too much, reduce the protein by a third.

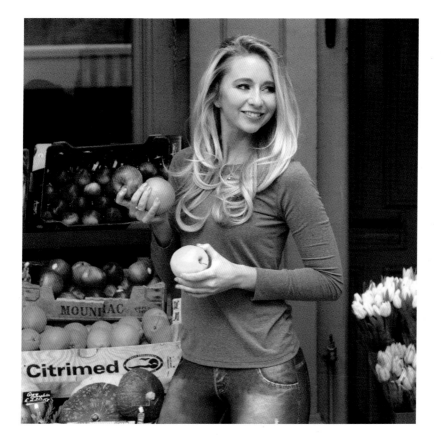

THE RE-NOURISH MENU

	BREAKFAST	LUNCH	DINNER	SNACKS/ DESSERTS
MONDAY (Meat free)	Porridge (choose from pages 120–1)	Sweet potato frittata A bowl of berries	Roasted vegetables with squash and tofu Polenta chips	4 oatcakes and/or 30g nut butter 1 apple
TUESDAY	Blueberry spinach smoothie	Buddha bowl	Black bean and mushroom chilli	Bowl of Greek or coconut yoghurt 2 satsumas
WEDNESDAY	Green and mean toast	Chicken and roasted vegetable skewers with Pesto butter beans	Salmon parcels Sweet potato and garlic purée	2 hard-boiled eggs Granola square
THURSDAY	Baked turmeric eggs	Baked potato with tuna mayo	Turkey tagine	25g mixed nuts Aubergine hummus (30g) and crudités
FRIDAY	Gingerbread breakfast biscuits	Mackerel cobb salad	Fish and chips or Crunchy cauliflower salad	Chocolate protein pancake
SATURDAY	Pistachio granola, plus 80g berries and 100g yoghurt	Courgette, pea and mint soup with rye bread	Sea bass with salsa verde and rice or simple green salad	Baked cinnamon apple with raisins
SUNDAY	The full healthy	Aubergine, feta and pomegranate salad	Quinoa-crusted macaroni cheese with a simple green salad or avocado and parsnip fries	Cacao yoghurt bowl

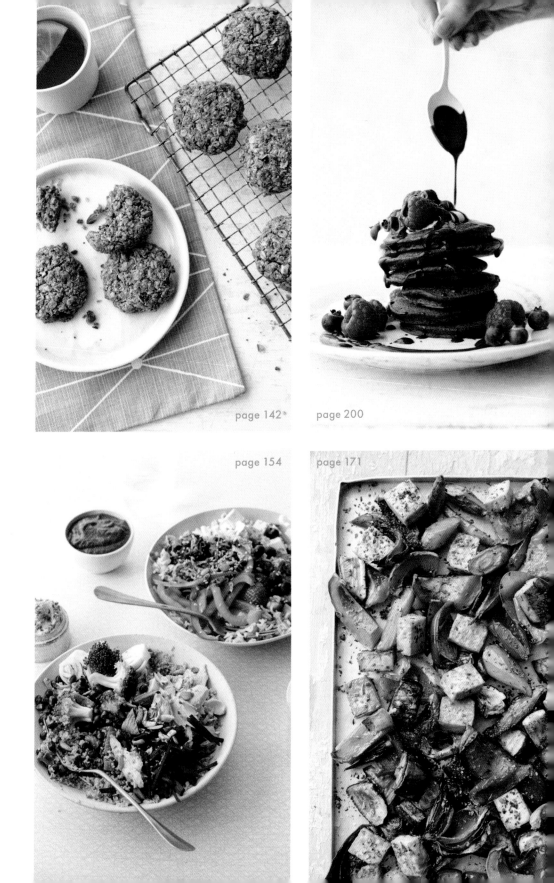

page 142

page 200

page 154

page 171

BREAKFAST

---◆---

In my eyes breakfast really is the most important meal of the day. In fact, when I wake up the first thing I do, after drinking some water, is to head to the kitchen and prepare my breakfast. Starting the morning off well really does set you up for a wonderfully energised day ahead – it's widely accepted that people who eat breakfast regularly feel healthier overall, have more energy and are typically leaner than those who don't eat in the morning. One of the keys to healthy eating is to start your day with a truly balanced breakfast that contains plenty of protein – an element that is often forgotten about first thing, yet is a key macronutrient that can help you stay fuller for longer. You'll find plenty of healthy options, both savoury and sweet, to keep you full and satisfied all the way until lunchtime.

The following recipes can be adapted for vegetarians or vegans and there are tasty options to make the night before, as well as items you can take with you on-the-go.

PORRIDGE 4 WAYS

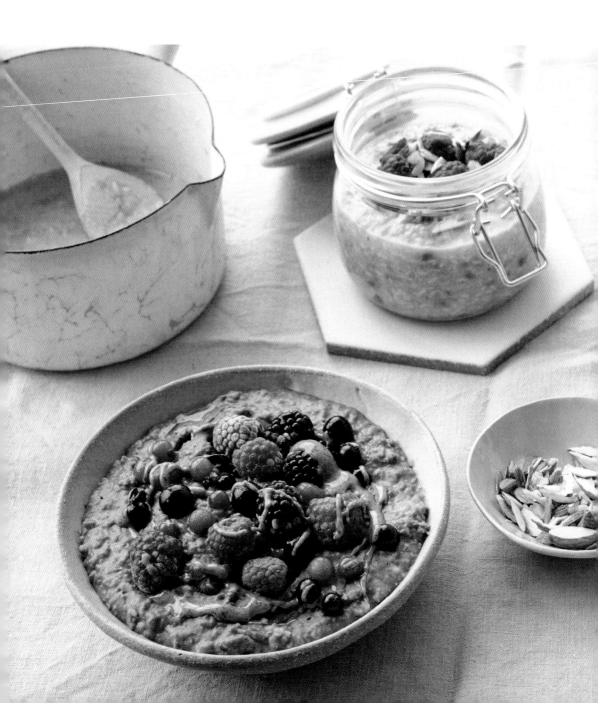

Porridge is my favourite breakfast. It never gets old, especially if you get creative with toppings. If made the right way, porridge will fill you up, providing you with a slow release of energy throughout the morning. For a more interesting porridge that will give you a boost of protein, try using quinoa flakes instead of oats; they also have the added advantage of cooking faster than traditional oats, in under 2 minutes – so that's less stirring time on the hob for you!

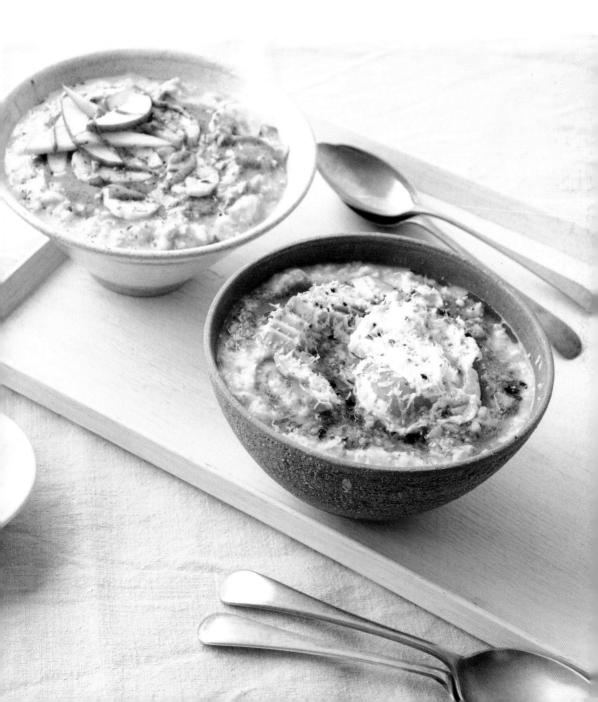

GRATED APPLE AND BANANA WITH CINNAMON

SERVES 1

50g rolled oats (or use jumbo oats)

½ apple, grated (keep the other half for your mid-morning snack or slice on top of the porridge)

1 small banana, thinly sliced

250ml milk of choice (I like hazelnut)

1 tsp ground cinnamon

15g nut butter (optional, for home-made see page 243)

I'm a massive apple crumble fan (in fact, I'm an anything-with-oats fan) so it's very easy to see where the inspiration for this porridge came from. You can make it the night before and leave it in the fridge – it makes an excellent overnight oats creation that you can take to work. I use porridge (also called rolled) oats as they cook really quickly. You can use jumbo oats here but they take longer to cook; you may also need more milk. And if you want an extra hit of protein try topping your porridge with a tablespoon of nut butter.

Put the oats, grated apple, half the sliced banana (reserve the rest for the top) and milk in a small pan. Stirring regularly, cook over a medium heat for 3–5 minutes until the porridge is creamy and has thickened.

Transfer to a bowl and top with the rest of the banana slices. Sprinkle over the cinnamon and top with nut butter, if using.

CACAO PORRIDGE WITH FROZEN BERRIES AND NUT BUTTER

SERVES 1

50g rolled oats

275ml milk of choice

1 scoop (30g) protein powder, your choice of flavour

1 tbsp raw cacao or unsweetened 100% cocoa powder

handful of frozen berries

15g nut butter (for home-made see page 243)

This is one of my favourite breakfasts, particularly as I always have cacao powder in my cupboard and frozen berries in my freezer. Frozen berries can actually be just as healthy as fresh – and in some cases more so – as fruits are generally picked at peak ripeness. This breakfast is so tasty you'll be amazed that it's actually good for you!

Put the oats, milk, protein powder and cacao or cocoa powder into a small pan. Stirring regularly, cook over a medium heat for 3–5 minutes until the porridge is creamy and has thickened. You may need to add more milk.

Transfer to a bowl and top with the berries and a drizzle of nut butter.

OVERNIGHT OATS
WITH RASPBERRIES AND COCONUT

SERVES 1

50g rolled oats

30g desiccated coconut

120ml coconut milk (from a tin if you prefer a thicker texture)

16 frozen raspberries, 10 roughly chopped and 6 left whole

handful of almonds, roughly chopped

If you're always in a rush in the morning, then this is the perfect solution as you can prepare this breakfast the night before. Make it in a jam jar for added convenience – just pop it into your bag the next day.

In a bowl or a jar with a tight-fitting lid, mix together the oats, coconut and coconut milk, then stir through the chopped raspberries. The oats should turn a nice pink colour. Cover (or add the lid) and leave in the fridge overnight.

If the oat mixture is too stiff in the morning, add a few tablespoons of water until you get the consistency you desire. Remove the whole raspberries from the freezer 5–10 minutes before you want to eat the oats. Top the oats with the raspberries and chopped almonds, and enjoy.

POACHED EGG AND AVOCADO

SERVES 1

50g rolled oats

1 tbsp pesto (optional)

1 egg

1 tbsp white vinegar (optional)

sprinkling of grated Parmesan

½ avocado, thinly sliced

pinch of cayenne pepper

salt and black pepper

Many years ago, when I was working as a steward at the Royal Albert Hall, a fellow redcoat told me that he put an egg in his porridge; I honestly laughed out loud but now I am totally hooked. It's almost like having a traditional breakfast, with oats replacing the bread.

Place the oats in a small pan with 250ml water and season with a pinch of salt and pepper. Warm over a medium heat, stirring frequently for about 3–5 minutes, until the water is absorbed and the oats are thickened. Stir in the pesto, if using.

To poach your egg, bring a pan of water to the boil. Turn to a gentle simmer and add the vinegar. Crack the egg into a small ramekin and gently ease the egg into the water. Cook for 3–4 minutes until the white is set and the yolk feels like the soft part of your cheek. Remove with a slotted spoon and drain on kitchen paper.

Transfer the cooked porridge to a bowl, top with the sliced avocado and your cooked egg and a sprinkle of freshly grated Parmesan. Garnish with a pinch of cayenne and some more black pepper.

I am a big fan of a healthy fry-up and I often mix up the ingredients, from vegetarian sausages to smoked salmon or tofu, so you can adapt this to suit all tastes. Broccoli contains many nutrients, including fibre, vitamins C and K, iron and potassium. It also contains more protein than most other vegetables so it's good to include wherever possible! My home-made Tomato Ketchup (see page 241) is great on the side too.

THE FULL HEALTHY

SERVES 2

olive oil, for frying

80g tenderstem broccoli

pinch of chilli flakes

100g spinach

1 lemon, quartered

160g halloumi, cut into 0.5cm thick slices

220g firm tofu, drained, patted dry with kitchen paper and crumbled (or use 120g smoked salmon)

pinch of ground turmeric

pinch of paprika

1 slice of rye bread per person (optional)

salt and black pepper

Heat 2 tablespoons of olive oil in a wok or a large frying pan over a medium-high heat. Add the broccoli and fry for 2–3 minutes, or until starting to soften, then stir in the chilli flakes. Next add the spinach, the juice from 1 lemon quarter and a pinch of salt to the pan and cook for 1–2 minutes until the spinach has wilted and the broccoli is tender. Move the veg to one side of the pan to make way for the tofu. (If you are using smoked salmon instead of tofu, skip the following step.)

Add a dash more olive oil to the pan and add the tofu with a pinch of salt and the turmeric. Cook, stirring, until lightly golden, which should take 3–4 minutes.

Meanwhile, in a small non-stick frying or griddle pan, warm a tablespoon of olive oil over a medium heat. Add the halloumi to the pan, sprinkle over the paprika and cook for 1–2 minutes on each side, or until browned. Meanwhile, toast the rye bread, if using.

Divide the cooked vegetables between two plates. Add the sliced tofu or smoked salmon, if using, and the fried halloumi slices. Season with a further sprinkle of chilli flakes and some black pepper and serve each plate with a wedge of lemon.

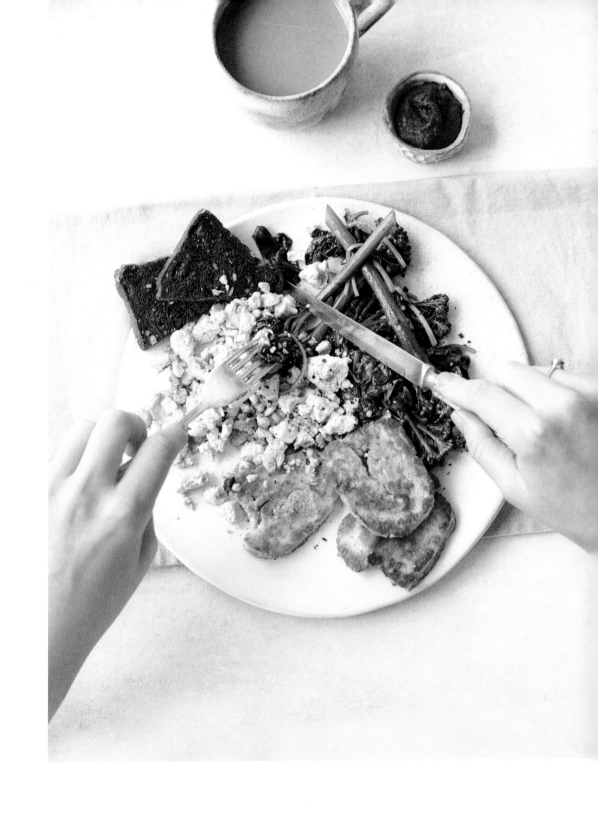

SMOOTHIE 4 WAYS

Smoothies are a great way to pack a nutrient punch and if you're in a rush you can drink on-the-go. On the following pages are four smoothies, each with their own special nutritional properties, so if you have a busy day ahead and are looking for a sharp mind, opt for the brain power smoothie; likewise if you are feeling a bit fragile, go for the happy tummy smoothie.

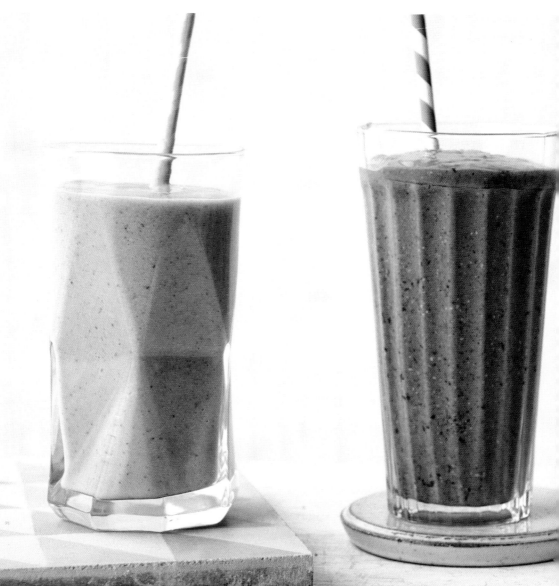

Almond Breakfast Smoothie
(healthy fats)

Happy Tummy Smoothie
(eases digestion)

Don't be scared to use frozen ingredients or to get creative with the recipe. If you don't like yoghurt, use quark or another source of protein such as cottage cheese or protein powder. Just make sure you have a high-speed blender able to blend frozen fruits or ice. The process for making all of my smoothies is the same: add all the ingredients to a blender and blitz until smooth – you always have the option to add more milk or water to reach the desired consistency. It's also a good idea to taste your smoothie before adding additional sweetener, such as honey. The recipes serve 1, but you can easily double them up.

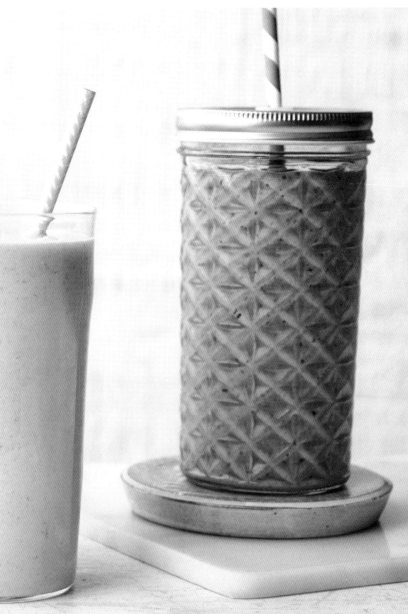

Zingy Orange Carrot Smoothie
(immunity)

Blueberry Spinach Smoothie
(brain power)

BLUEBERRY SPINACH SMOOTHIE (BRAIN POWER)

SERVES 1 (MAKES 500ML)

125ml milk of choice

135g Greek yoghurt

125g frozen blueberries

1 large frozen strawberry

½ ripe banana

25g spinach

1 scoop (25–30g) protein powder (optional)

½ tbsp honey, or to taste (optional)

Blueberries are super-good for us: low in calories, high in fibre and full of vitamin C, vitamin K and manganese. Blueberries have the highest antioxidant capacity of all commonly consumed fruits and vegetables. These antioxidants are called flavonoids and may help to improve brain function and delay age-related cognitive decline.

Blend all the ingredients together, adding more milk to thin or honey to sweeten, as needed.

ZINGY ORANGE CARROT SMOOTHIE (IMMUNITY)

SERVES 1 (MAKES 450ML)

150g yoghurt of choice (vanilla, natural or dairy-free)

handful of ice cubes

1 medium carrot (about 80g), roughly chopped (grate the carrot if you don't have a high-speed blender)

1 large orange, peeled

small chunk of fresh ginger (or use 1 tsp ground ginger)

30g rolled oats

2 tbsp hemp seeds or ground flaxseeds

pinch of salt

1 tbsp honey (optional)

Keep your energy high with this fibre-rich smoothie. Anything orange is often a good source of beta-carotene (which is converted to vitamin A) and vitamin C. Carrots are also a good source of several B vitamins, vitamin K and potassium so will do more for you than just help you see in the dark! Keep sickness away with this immune-boosting breakfast.

Add all the ingredients except the honey to a blender with 250ml water and blend until smooth. Taste for sweetness and add honey if desired.

HAPPY TUMMY SMOOTHIE (EASES DIGESTION)

SERVES 1 (MAKES 500ML)

165ml coconut water (or use a plant-based milk)

1 small avocado, peeled and stoned (about 80g avocado flesh)

handful of frozen pineapple chunks (about 60g)

½ medium banana, sliced and frozen

handful of parsley leaves (about 5g)

2 tsp ground flaxseeds (optional)

1 tsp grated ginger (if you have a high-speed blender throw in a whole thumb-sized chunk, unpeeled)

juice of 1–2 limes

1–2 sprigs of fresh mint (optional)

There are lots of claims when it comes to foods that help aid digestion. Pineapples contain the enzyme bromelain, which has been shown to decrease inflammation and stimulate the immune system. But it is also linked to a healthy digestion, which, when coupled with ginger, banana, parsley and avocado is good for our tummies!

Add the ingredients to a blender with 165ml water and blend until smooth.

Add more water or coconut water if you prefer a thinner smoothie.

ALMOND BREAKFAST SMOOTHIE (HEALTHY FATS)

SERVES 1 (MAKES 500ML)

250ml almond milk

120g frozen raspberries (or use a combination of raspberries, strawberries, blueberries etc.)

1 medium banana, sliced and frozen

30g rolled oats

1 scoop (25–30g) protein powder (I like vanilla in this smoothie)

1 tbsp almond butter

1 tsp ground cinnamon

I love this smoothie as it's so thick and creamy. Almonds are rich in healthy monounsaturated fats, fibre and protein; they are also one of the best sources of Vitamin E, which protects your cell membranes from damage, contributing towards healthy skin and a healthy heart.

Blend all the ingredients together. This smoothie is quite thick. If you prefer a thinner consistency, add more a little more milk.

There is absolutely nothing wrong with bread as long as you choose wisely. Opt for a wholegrain variety that will keep you fuller for longer and provide you with gut-friendly fibre over any white bread. Or why not go for sourdough, or a dense rye full of seeds and grains? If you are avoiding gluten there are still plenty of readily available options, but please read the label and check for added calories and sugars. In fact, a good slice of toast can be the basis for a speedy and healthy meal at any time of the day – if you know what to put on it. The recipes on the following pages all serve 1 but can easily be doubled up.

TOAST 4 WAYS

GREEN AND MEAN

SERVES 1

1 slice of bread

½ ripe avocado

50g cooked and shelled edamame beans

handful of watercress

salt and black pepper

olive oil and toasted seeds, to serve (optional)

Edamame beans are a fabulous source of protein – they are around 12 per cent protein, which is a decent amount for a plant food. They are also a complete protein, making them a good source of all essential amino acids.

Toast the bread while you mash the avocado; season with salt and pepper and then spread over the bread. Top with the edamame beans and watercress and finish with a drizzle of olive oil and some toasted seeds, if liked.

SARDINES ON TOAST

SERVES 1

1 slice of bread

3 sardines in olive oil

5 cherry tomatoes, halved or quartered

20–25g walnuts, roughly chopped

drizzle of balsamic vinegar and a few torn basil leaves, to serve (optional)

Sardines are one of those brilliant store-cupboard staples: they're cheap, last for ages and give us SO much nutrition! They are one of the few edible sources of vitamin D and calcium, thanks to their soft bones – not forgetting the amazing omega-3 fatty acids!

Toast the bread and then top with the sardines. Mash them in with a fork. Add the tomatoes and walnuts and finish with a drizzle of balsamic vinegar and some torn basil, if using.

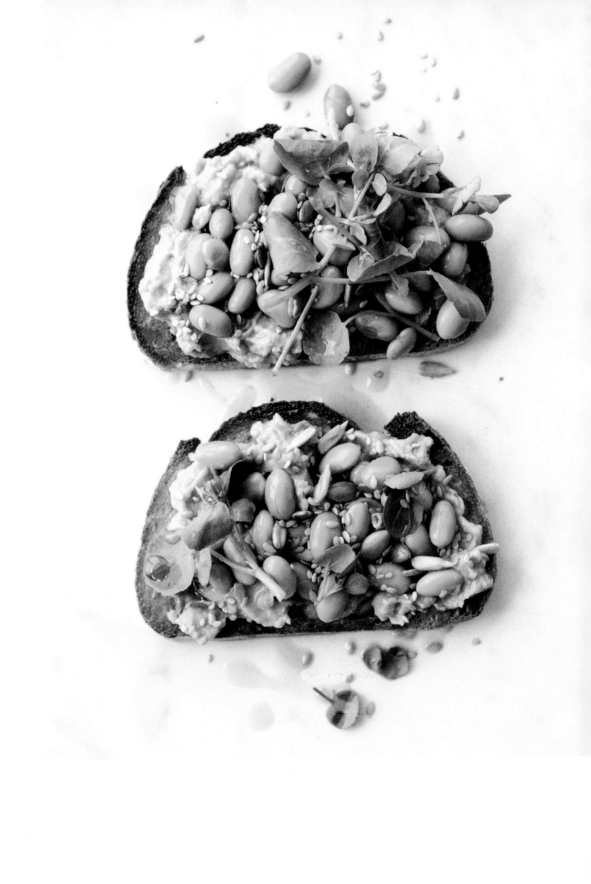

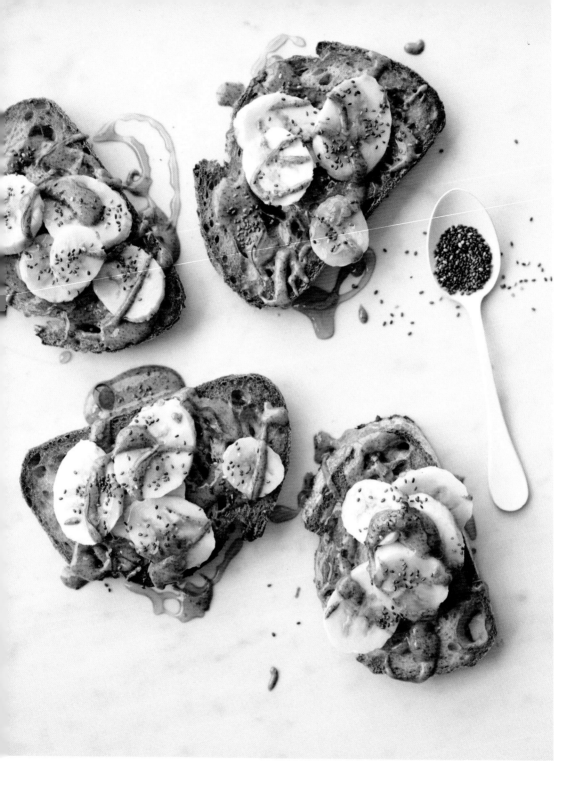

PEAR AND CHEESE

SERVES 1

1 slice of bread

100g cottage cheese or 40g feta, crumbled

1 small pear, peeled, cored and thinly sliced

toasted seeds, olive oil and honey, to serve (optional)

This topping is inspired by my late grandparents' love for traditional sandwiches and salads. I picked two of their favourite things – cheese and pears – and have created this super scrumptious topping for you. The natural sweetness from the pear really does make this breakfast feel like a treat! You can also try this with figs when they are in season.

Toast the bread and top with the cheese. Arrange the sliced pear on the top.

Scatter with toasted seeds and drizzle with a little olive oil and honey, if liked.

BANANA TOAST

SERVES 1

1 slice of bread

1 heaped tbsp nut butter, (for home-made see page 243)

1 medium banana, sliced

1–2 tsp chia seeds (or any seeds you like)

honey or maple syrup, to drizzle (optional)

I often see people adding banana to their toast but then forgetting the crucial macronutrient at breakfast – protein! I have paired the banana with some nut butter and chia seeds to boost the protein content but if you're not a fan of nuts try adding some hemp seeds.

Toast the bread and spread with the nut butter.

Add the sliced banana and sprinkle with seeds. Serve with a drizzle of honey or maple syrup, if liked.

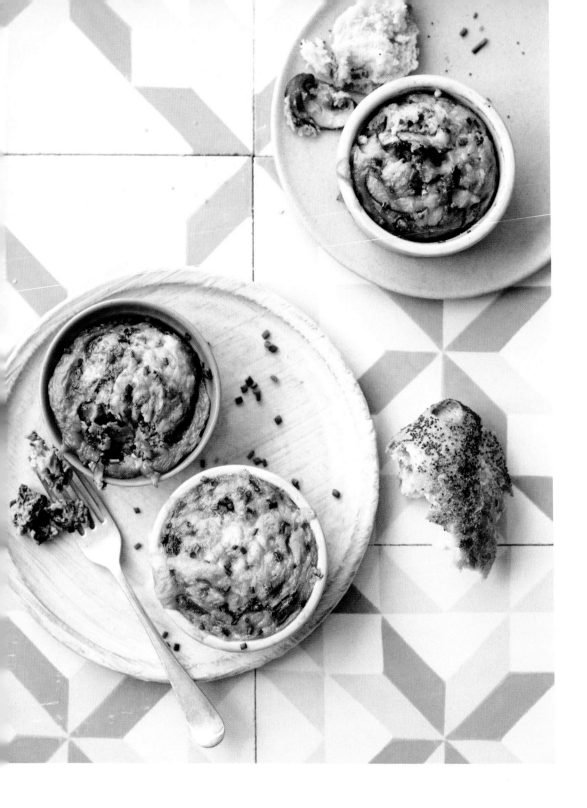

I believe in using what's in the spice cupboard at every opportunity. One of the simplest ways to use turmeric is to add its distinct yellow colour to your eggs. Curcumin is the main active ingredient in turmeric; it's said to have powerful anti-inflammatory effects and is a very strong antioxidant. Be aware that you do need a large amount of turmeric to see the benefits that some of the studies report – add a pinch of black pepper to aid absorption. This recipe is delicious and works well whether you use one, two or all three of the suggested filling ingredients. Double up the recipe if you are serving more people.

BAKED TURMERIC EGGS

SERVES 1

1 tsp ground turmeric

2 medium eggs

1 tbsp grated hard cheese or 2 tbsp soft cheese, such as cottage cheese (optional)

handful of herbs, such as chives or parsley, chopped, (optional)

pinch of salt and black pepper

Filling options

20g spinach, shredded

1 tomato, diced

1–2 mushrooms, thinly sliced

Preheat the oven to 200°C fan/220°C/425°F/gas mark 7.

Lightly grease 2 small ovenproof ramekins (capacity 150ml) or small baking dishes with a little oil or butter and then divide your prepped chosen fillings between the ramekins.

Whisk together the turmeric with the eggs then stir in the cheese and herbs, if using. Season with salt and pepper and pour into the ramekins over your fillings.

Bake for 12–15 minutes until the egg is browned and set on top.

Curry powder is a fab way of adding spice (rather than heat) to your food. You can leave out the fresh chilli if you prefer less heat. Kedgeree is a classic Indian rice dish that became popular in the UK in various guises but ultimately it consists of rice, smoked haddock, eggs and curry powder. Haddock is an extremely nutritious fish, high in protein and low in fat so it's ideal if you're looking to include a variety of fish in your diet; swap the fish for tofu for a vegetarian option. I've also switched the white rice for wholegrain rice or quinoa to up the fibre and protein content.

SMOKED HADDOCK (OR TOFU) KEDGEREE

SERVES 4

170g wholegrain rice or quinoa

4 medium eggs

500g undyed smoked haddock (or mackerel) fillets, from sustainable sources if possible (or use 250g firm tofu, drained and cubed)

2 bay leaves

1 tbsp butter (or coconut oil)

1 onion, finely chopped (or use 1 bunch of spring onions)

1 garlic clove, very finely chopped

1 thumb-sized piece of fresh ginger, peeled and grated

2 tbsp curry powder

2 large beef tomatoes or 4 salad tomatoes, deseeded and cut into small dice

2 lemons

First cook your rice or quinoa in boiling salted water until soft, but still retaining some bite. Depending on the grain you use it will take between 15–25 minutes so check the instructions on the packet. Drain and refresh in cold water, then set aside until ready to use.

While the rice is cooking, hard-boil the eggs: put them into a pan, cover with cold water and place over a high heat. When the water comes to the boil, add a lid, remove from the heat and leave to stand for 10 minutes. (You can boil the eggs any way you like; this is just how I like to do it.) Drain and cool the eggs by refreshing under cold water. When they are cool enough to handle, peel and cut into quarters.

Next cook your fish. Put the fish in a single layer in a wide shallow pan, pour over enough water to cover the fish and add your bay leaves. Bring to the boil, cover and simmer for about 5 minutes, until the fish is opaque and flakes easily. Remove the fish from the pan, discard any skin and flake the flesh into chunks; set aside.

When you have prepared the rice, eggs and fish you are ready to finish off the dish. Melt the butter in a large frying pan over a low heat. Add the onion with a pinch of salt and cook until softened, about 5 minutes. Next add the garlic and ginger and sauté for another minute before adding the curry powder. Allow the spices to toast in the heat

2 handfuls of coriander, roughly chopped

1 small fresh red chilli, very finely chopped (or use 1 tbsp chilli flakes)

salt and black pepper

250g natural yoghurt (or use dairy-free coconut yoghurt), to serve

of the pan for a few more minutes before adding the diced tomatoes and the juice of 1 of the lemons.

Add the rice to the pan and toss to coat in the spices, then gently fold in the flaked fish (or the cubed tofu) and the eggs, then finally most of the chopped coriander and chilli. Season to taste with salt and black pepper.

Mix the remaining chopped coriander into the yoghurt, and serve this and the other lemon, cut into quarters, with the kedgeree.

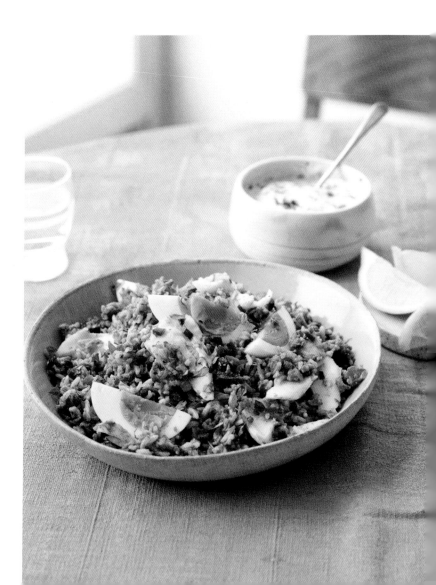

This is one of those recipes that most of my clients turn their noses up at, but once they try it, they're hooked. Don't let the colour put you off; in fact, embrace that vibrant green. This is an easy way of getting vegetables into your diet first thing, starting the day with a burst of micronutrients.

GREEN SMOOTHIE BOWL

SERVES 1

150ml milk of choice (I like almond or coconut)

20g oats or quinoa flakes

1 scoop (30g) vanilla protein powder or 100g Greek yoghurt

½ avocado

¼ cucumber

15 frozen grapes (I always keep a punnet in the freezer)

handful of spinach leaves

handful of mint leaves

2.5cm piece of fresh ginger

chopped almonds, mixed seeds or 1 tbsp home-made granola (see opposite), to top

Place all the ingredients (apart from the toppings) in a high-speed blender and blend until completely smooth. It will be thicker than a normal smoothie.

Pour into a bowl and sprinkle with chopped almonds, seeds or my Pistachio Granola, if you wish. Eat with a spoon!

Granola is one of my all-time favourite breakfasts – I just love the crunch! My issue with packets that you find in the supermarkets is that they are often full of extra sugar. But granola doesn't have to be unhealthy. My recipe is sweetened with stevia but you can use honey or maple syrup for extra taste. I've used my favourite nuts; those tasty pistachios are one of the better nuts for protein content per gram and are lower in saturated fat than others. Serve with milk of your choice or 150g Greek yoghurt and fresh fruit if you like.

PISTACHIO GRANOLA

MAKES 600G (12 X 50G SERVINGS)

75g coconut oil

2 tbsp honey (or use maple syrup)

100g jumbo oats (or use quinoa/buckwheat flakes)

70g pistachio nuts, chopped or left whole

60g sunflower seeds

50g pumpkin seeds

30g coconut flakes

1 tsp ground cinnamon

¼ tsp ground nutmeg

¼ tsp sea salt

2 tbsp cacao powder (optional, for a chocolate kick)

Preheat the oven to 180°C fan/200°C/400°F/gas mark 6 and line a baking tray with baking paper.

Melt the coconut oil and honey in a small pan, stirring well. Meanwhile put all the dry ingredients into a bowl and mix well.

Pour the coconut oil and honey over the dry ingredients and stir until all the oats are covered in the wet mix.

Spread evenly over the baking tray and bake in the middle shelf of the oven for 10 minutes. Remove, stir the granola and bake for another 5 minutes until the granola is browned all over. Watch it carefully as not all ovens bake at the same speed.

Who says salads are just for lunch and dinner? This one is delicious and contains my favourite fruit – figs, which contain both fibre and calcium. Salads can be balanced too, and this will leave you feeling satisfied and full all morning. You'll have also had a massive injection of nutrition from the variety of ingredients.

GREEN BREAKFAST SALAD

SERVES 1

50g salad leaves

½ avocado or
10 green olives

1 tomato, chopped

1 dried fig, sliced or finely chopped (or use a handful of sliced strawberries or sliced green grapes)

10g roasted hazelnuts, chopped

1 tbsp whole flaxseeds

2 hard- or soft-boiled medium eggs
(or use 100g cooked tofu)

juice of ½ lemon

salt and black pepper

rye bread, to serve
(optional)

Arrange the salad leaves in your bowl and build up your salad with the avocado or olives, tomato, fruit, nuts, seeds and cooked eggs or tofu.

Squeeze over the lemon juice and season with a pinch of salt and pepper. Toss gently and serve with rye bread.

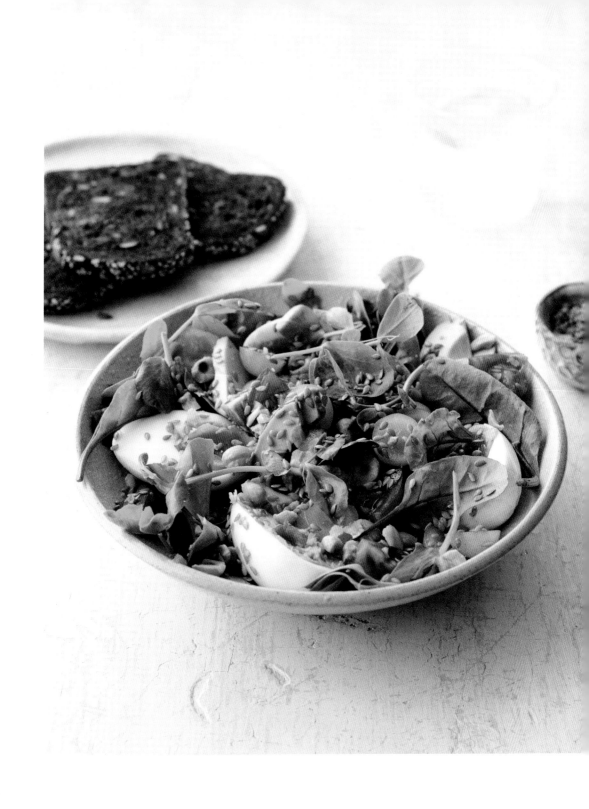

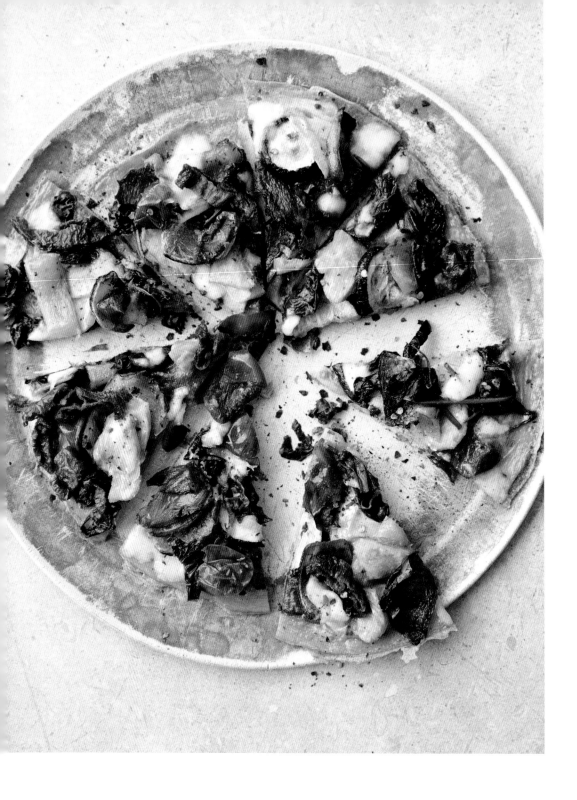

This has to be one of my signature breakfasts; it's honestly super-easy and so satisfying. You can really get creative here and turn this into your own favourite healthy breakfast. Boost the nutritional value by making your rainbow omelette as colourful as possible and don't be scared to try new toppings. In terms of your vegetable intake, the saying 'eat a rainbow' really does make sense and it's worth thinking about how to add in more colour whenever you can! Serve with a few salad leaves or a slice of rye bread.

RAINBOW PIZZA OMELETTE

SERVES 2

5 medium eggs

¼ tsp ground turmeric (optional)

½ tsp chilli flakes

1 tbsp olive oil

80g roasted vegetables (about 1 aubergine or 1 courgette or 1–2 peppers)

60g tuna or salmon, flaked (fresh or tinned)

30g mozzarella, torn

handful of cooked kale or raw spinach leaves

4 sun-dried tomatoes, chopped

salt and black pepper

Preheat the oven to 180°C fan/200°C/400°F/gas mark 6.

Whisk the eggs in a small bowl with the turmeric and chilli flakes and season with salt and pepper.

Heat the oil in a medium ovenproof frying pan over a low heat. Pour in the eggs, swirl around the pan, and then leave to cook over a low heat for 5 minutes. Transfer to the preheated oven and cook for 2–3 minutes until the top starts to brown.

Remove from the oven, scatter over your toppings and return to the oven for another 3 minutes until the cheese has melted and the top of the omelette is set.

If you have a family you may sometimes find it hard to get everyone to eat breakfast in the morning. These biscuits are a lovely, healthy home-made alternative to the usual breakfast staples. Oats are such a good heart-healthy ingredient to include in your diet, with well documented benefits, from weight loss to reduced blood sugar levels and a reduced risk of heart disease.

GINGERBREAD BREAKFAST BISCUITS

SERVES 8

80g coconut oil

75ml honey

60ml almond milk

2 tsp vanilla extract

100g rolled oats

35g desiccated coconut

25g ground almonds

15g nuts of your choice, chopped

1 tbsp chia seeds

2cm piece of fresh ginger, peeled and grated or ½ tsp ground ginger (or use both if you love it!)

1 tsp ground cinnamon

pinch of sea salt

Preheat the oven to 180°C fan/200°C/400°F/gas mark 6 and line a baking tray with baking paper.

Melt the coconut oil in a small pan, then remove from the heat and add the honey, almond milk and vanilla extract. Stir well.

Meanwhile, mix together all the dry ingredients in a large bowl so they are well combined. Pour the wet ingredients into the bowl, stir well and leave for 10 minutes for the chia seeds to expand (this helps the biscuits stick together).

After 10 minutes use wet hands to scoop and shape the mixture into 8 even-sized balls on your baking tray. Flatten them with a fork and smoothly shape the edges with your fingertips.

Bake for 15–18 minutes until browned all over. Remove from the oven and allow to cool fully before eating. The biscuits will still be quite soft but will harden as they cool.

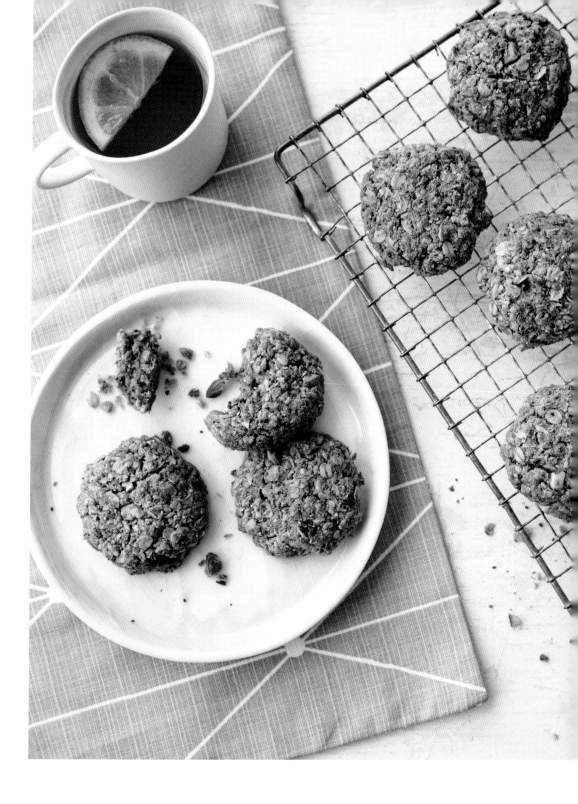

LUNCH

I rarely have time to make glamorous lunches and, let's face it, most of us are constantly running from A to B during the day. But that doesn't mean we have to compromise on taste and nutrition. I have created some really delicious lunch options, varying from super-speedy and portable to things to enjoy on those days when you have a bit more time. Lunches should always be balanced and tailored to your needs – I believe in colourful vegetables bursting full of micronutrients and fibre paired with protein, healthy fats and carbohydrates to give you the best possible fuel for the afternoon. From salads to hot and cold dishes, you can really keep it varied. Invest in some decent Tupperware and you can take any meal with you – just don't forget your knife and fork! Be mindful that variety is key when it comes to a healthy body and mind, so don't get stuck in the rut of eating the same every day. Mix it up!

Frittatas are super-satisfying; they feel like such a treat to have at any time of day. They also make a great on-the-go option as you can serve them cold; just make the night before and you can divide into sections and take to work in a lunchbox. My favourite combination is sweet potato with feta cheese but you can also add other items to it. Spinach, kale or greens make a really nice addition and add texture, but perhaps lightly wilt them for a few minutes in a pan with some olive oil and a pinch of salt. Perfection!

SWEET POTATO FRITTATA

SERVES 3–4

1 large sweet potato

1 tbsp olive oil

2 red onions, thinly sliced

2 small garlic cloves, very finely chopped

6 large eggs

100g feta

pinch of ground nutmeg

handful of parsley, finely chopped (optional)

salt and black pepper

salad leaves, to serve

Preheat the oven to 190°C fan/210°C/420°F/gas mark 6½.

Prick the sweet potato with a fork a few times and bake whole for 40 minutes, or until cooked through. Remove and set aside to cool.

While the sweet potatoes are baking, heat the oil in a 26cm ovenproof frying pan over a low-medium heat. Add the onions with a pinch of salt and cook for 10 minutes, until soft, stirring regularly (if you use a lid they will soften more quickly). Add the garlic and cook for a further minute.

Meanwhile crack the eggs into a bowl, crumble in the cheese, add the nutmeg and seasoning and whisk. Add the chopped parsley, if using (reserve a little to scatter on at the end).

When both the onions and sweet potatoes are ready, scoop out the sweet potato flesh, discarding the skins, and dollop evenly around the pan on top of the onions. Pour the egg mixture over and cook over a medium heat for 5 minutes until the eggs start to set around the edges of the pan.

Transfer to the oven and cook for 10–12 minutes, or until cooked through and browned on top. If you like a really browned top, slide the pan under a hot grill. Serve hot, warm or cold, scattered with the reserved parsley, if using, and with a few salad leaves alongside.

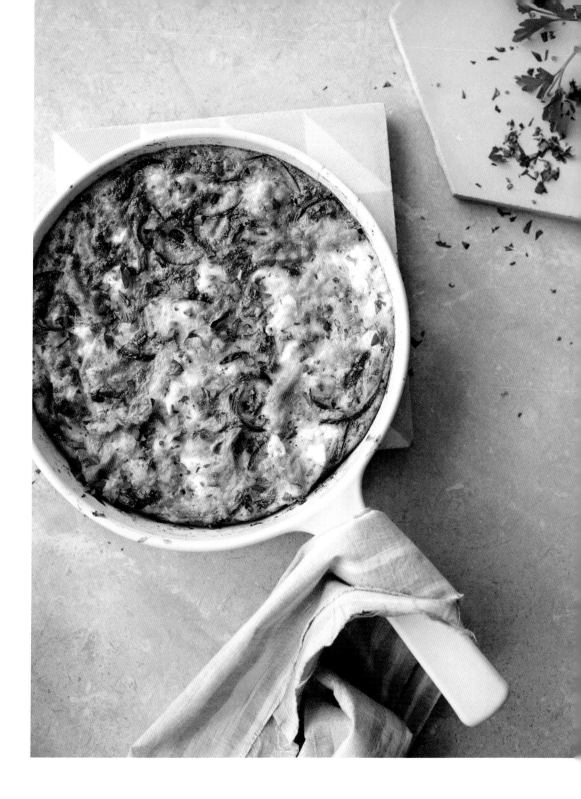

If you are getting bored of the same old lunches, give my burritos a try. These can be fun to make and you can customise them to include your favourite food combinations. Use regular wholemeal or multigrain wraps – although in some supermarkets you can now find new and exciting wraps made from quinoa or sweet potato.

Decide which protein filling you want to use, follow the recipe and then build your perfect burrito using whatever you like from the suggestions listed opposite. You can boost the veg content or even make a lighter version with large lettuce leaves!

If you want to eat this at work I'd suggest you transport your wrap and fillings separately – that way you'll get a nice fresh burrito and not a soggy one by the time lunch comes around.

BURRITOS

SERVES 2

4 tortilla wraps (or use 4 large lettuce leaves)

For the grains (optional)

120g brown rice or quinoa

60g tinned sweetcorn

For the base

1 tbsp olive oil

2 white onions, thinly sliced

1 garlic clove, very finely chopped

For the protein filling (choose one)

1 x 400g tin black beans, drained and rinsed

350g chicken breast, sliced into strips

350g sirloin steak, sliced into strips

½ aubergine, cubed, plus 200g firm tofu, cut into 2.5cm slices

If you are adding grains to your burrito, cook them according to the packet instructions. Drain and refresh in cold water, then mix with the sweetcorn and set aside.

To make your base, put the olive oil into a medium frying pan and place over a medium heat. Add the onions and sauté for 3–4 minutes until softened, before stirring in the garlic.

Next add your chosen filling ingredient, plus the spices and a pinch of salt and pepper. Each filling has a different cooking time: beans will need around 10 minutes; chicken strips 10–12 minutes; steak strips about 5 minutes; the aubergine will need a good 10 minutes before you add the tofu and cook for a further 5 minutes.

Now add your additional veg, such as peppers or mushrooms. Cook for a further 5 minutes, stirring regularly. Squeeze over the lime juice, taste and adjust the seasoning if necessary.

For the spices

2 tsp paprika

1 tsp cayenne pepper

pinch of chilli flakes

salt and black pepper

For the extra veg

2–3 peppers (any colour), deseeded and thinly sliced

150g mushrooms, quartered

1 tbsp lime juice

For the extras (optional)

1 avocado, mashed

1 jalapeño chilli, very finely chopped

1 tbsp Greek yoghurt

handful of grated cheese

handful of coriander, chopped

Get your burrito extras prepped in separate bowls so you are ready to build your perfect burrito. Place the filling in a line down the middle of the wrap and top with any extras. Fold one side of the wrap over the filling, and then fold the two outer edges in before folding the other so that none of your lovely filling escapes!

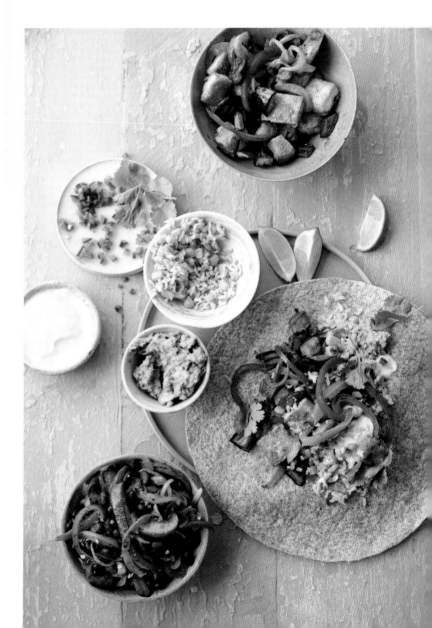

Sandwiches have had a bit of bad rep lately. Bread and carb deniers often label them as an unhealthy choices but it certainly doesn't have to be that way if you fill them with good stuff! These are both protein-packed options, but they are also balanced, so you're getting a variety of vitamins and minerals. Not to mention these are also more exciting than your usual ham and cheese (although if that's what you fancy, go for it). I use rye bread as it's nice and firm, full of fibre and can take heavy toppings, but feel free to use sourdough or wholegrain bread.

SMØRREBRØD (DANISH OPEN SANDWICH)

SERVES 2

2 slices of rye bread

100g ricotta

coconut oil, olive oil or butter, for frying

1 garlic clove, very finely chopped

60g spinach leaves

2 medium eggs

black pepper

EGG AND RICOTTA FLORENTINE

This is such a simple recipe yet it tastes so satisfying. Never underestimate the power of cheese and eggs. This will provide you with some vitamin D, calcium and plenty of protein.

Preheat the oven to 180°C fan/200°C/400°F/gas mark 6.

Place the slices of bread on a baking tray and spread the ricotta over the top. Bake for 6–8 minutes – this will warm the bread and slightly brown the cheese.

Meanwhile, add a tablespoon of oil or butter to a frying pan, and when warm add the garlic and sauté for around 30 seconds. Next add the spinach leaves and cook until they wilt down, about 2 minutes. Drain the garlicky spinach on kitchen paper while you cook your eggs. If the pan is dry add a little more oil and then fry your eggs until the white is set.

Remove the ricotta-topped rye slices from the oven, transfer to two plates and heap the garlicky spinach and a fried egg on top of each one. Season liberally with black pepper.

SERVES 2

2 slices of rye bread

40g goat's cheese

2 slices of prosciutto

1 fig, sliced

salad leves, to garnish

balsamic vinegar, for drizzling

black pepper

FIG AND PROSCIUTTO

My favourite fruit, figs, always remind me of times on holiday in Italy, eating antipasti of figs paired with prosciutto in the sunshine. This combination of sweet and savoury works so well.

Lightly toast the bread, then spread the goat's cheese on top of each piece. Top with the prosciutto, sliced fig, and salad leaves, to garnish. Drizzle with balsamic vinegar and season with black pepper.

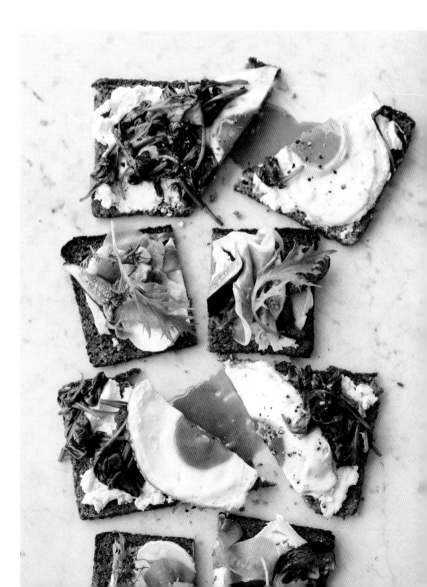

Aubergine is my all-time favourite vegetable – I am addicted to its texture when it's cooked well. Aubergine also contains an antioxidant known as nasunin, in the purple pigment of its skin. Researchers have reported that nasunin helps reduce free radicals and may protect brain health. I am so excited to share my favourite salad with you – it's so delicious and the combination of colour, taste and texture ticks all the boxes. Pomegranate seeds are an excellent addition to salads and main dishes so buy them whenever they're on offer.

AUBERGINE, FETA AND POMEGRANATE SALAD

SERVES 2

2 small aubergines, diced into 3cm chunks

olive oil

150g green leaves (I like a mix of spinach, lettuce, rocket and parsley leaves)

8 cherry tomatoes, halved

6 dried apricots, cut into chunks

juice of ½ lemon

60g feta, crumbled

100g pomegranate seeds

handful of chopped roasted hazelnuts (about 20g)

salt and black pepper

Preheat the oven to 160°C fan/180°C/350°F/gas mark 4.

Arrange the aubergine chunks in a single layer in a roasting tray. Sprinkle with a good pinch of salt and pepper and a couple of glugs of olive oil (about 1–2 tablespoons). Toss to ensure the aubergine is coated well then roast for 30–40 minutes, stirring halfway cooking, until golden.

While the aubergine is roasting, place the green leaves, cherry tomatoes and chopped apricots in a mixing bowl and toss with 2 tablespoons of olive, the lemon juice and a pinch of salt and pepper.

Remove the roasted aubergine from the oven, allow to cool for 3–5 minutes, then add to the salad bowl; its heat should wilt the leaves a little.

Add the feta and sprinkle over the pomegranates and chopped hazelnuts. Finish with an extra drizzle of olive oil if you like.

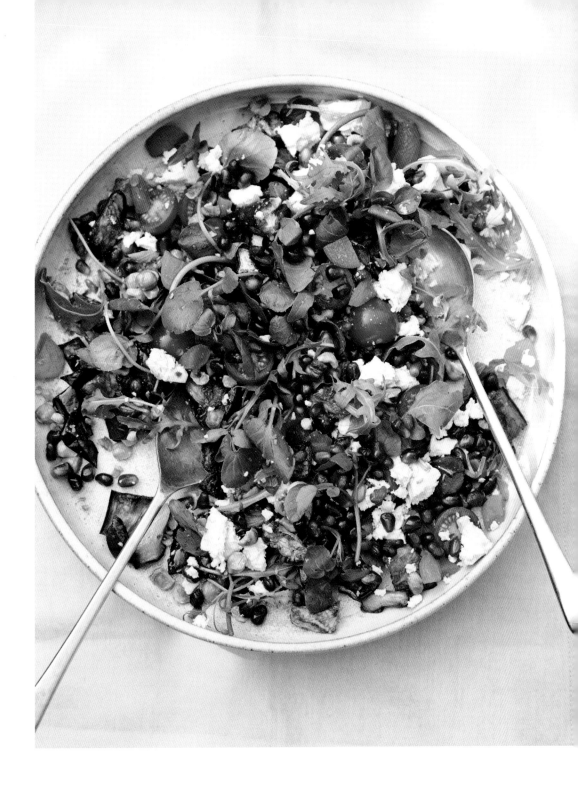

Healthy doesn't have to mean complicated or unsatisfying. My Buddha bowls are hearty, filling dishes packed with greens, raw or roasted veg, optional fruit, a portion of protein and a healthy grain like quinoa or brown rice. The best bit is you can choose depending on the ingredients you have to hand. Simply pick one green base for your bowl, mix it in with your choice of healthy grains, add a protein, two or three vegetable options (depending on how hungry you are) and three toppings. And if you want a low-carb option just double up on the greens and leave out the grains. Simple!

BUILD YOUR BUDDHA BOWL

SERVES 2

CHOOSE YOUR GREENS	CHOOSE A PROTEIN	CHOOSE A DIP (SEE PAGES 233–5)	CHOOSE YOUR TOPPINGS
200g combination of kale and spinach, roughly chopped and wilted in a frying pan with 1 tbsp oil 250g combination of broccoli and pak choi, steamed 200g combination of cabbage and cavolo nero, shredded and steamed	150g firm tofu, cubed and sautéed 150g cooked chicken, shredded or sliced 150g tinned or cooked fish, flaked	Aubergine Hummus Tzatziki Beetroot Dip Pea and Mint Purée	1 fresh or dried fig, diced 50g pomegranate seeds 40g blueberries 40g strawberries, chopped 1 tbsp seeds, toasted 1 tbsp chopped pistachios, toasted 1 tbsp flaked almonds, toasted Drizzle of olive oil
	CHOOSE YOUR VEGETABLES	**CHOOSE YOUR GRAINS**	
	80g carrot, grated 80g raw beetroot, grated 80g peppers, thinly sliced 200g roasted vegetables	60–80g quinoa, cooked 60–80g brown rice, cooked 160g polenta, cooked	

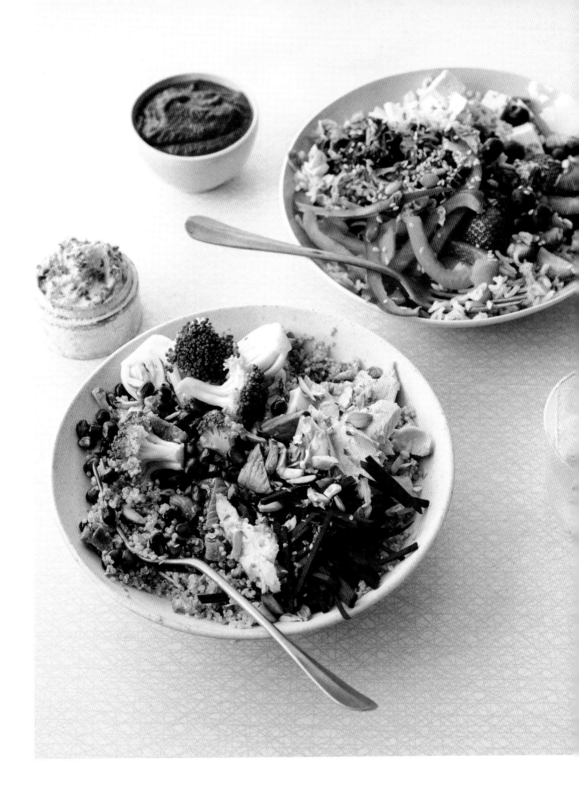

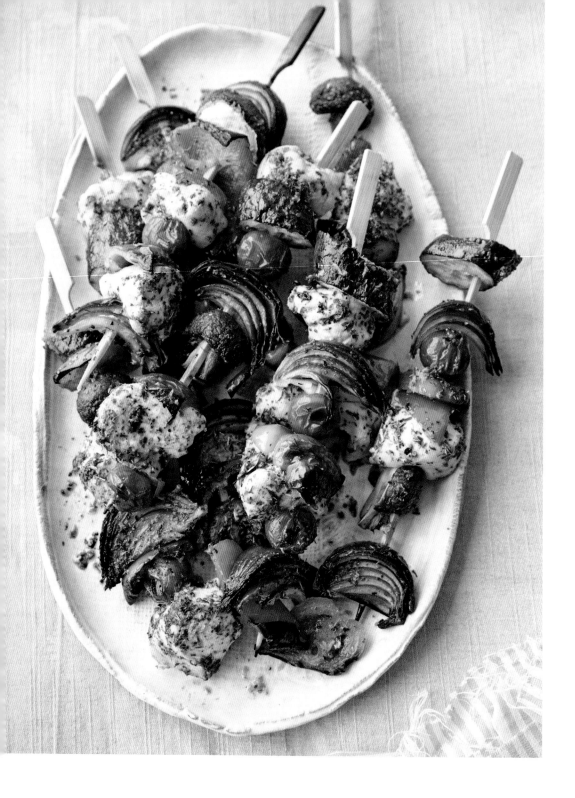

If you need an easy meal that is quick to make then look no further! This colourful option contains masses of vitamins and minerals with the added bonus that the skewers can be prepared in advance too. You can serve these with any of the dips on pages 232–5, and I often serve these with the Cucumber Tabbouleh (see page 163) for a refreshing side dish. Don't forget these can be eaten hot or cold, which make them ideal to take to work.

CHICKEN AND ROASTED VEGETABLE SKEWERS

SERVES 4

For the marinade

3 tbsp olive oil

4 tbsp lemon juice

2 tbsp dried oregano

3 garlic cloves, very finely chopped

salt and black pepper

For the skewers

4 chicken breasts, cut into 4cm cubes

1 courgette, cut into chunks

1 red pepper, deseeded and cut into 3cm pieces

1 green pepper, deseeded and cut into 3cm pieces

8 cherry tomatoes

5 mushrooms (any large ones, halved)

1 red onion, cut into wedges

8 long wooden skewers, soaked in water for 30 minutes

First make up your marinade by whisking all of the ingredients together, with a pinch of salt and pepper, in a small bowl until well combined.

Take two ziplock bags or Tupperware containers and put the chicken in one and all the vegetables in the other. Split the marinade between the bags or containers and seal. Make sure all of the ingredients are well coated in the marinade. Allow to marinate for at least 30 minutes and up to a maximum of overnight (in the fridge).

Meanwhile, preheat the oven to 180°C fan/200°C/400°F/gas mark 6 and line a baking tray with foil or baking paper.

Thread the chicken and vegetables evenly on to the skewers and lay them on the baking tray. Reserve any marinade for basting.

Roast for 15 minutes, then turn over and baste with any remaining marinade. Cook for a further 15 minutes until the chicken is cooked through.

This is a beautiful and vibrant soup that will boost your vegetable intake for the day. I don't see many people taking flasks to work these days and I think it's a real shame; home-made soup is such a fabulous lunchtime option and is a great way to save some pennies! Reheating this soup is perfectly fine as long as you heat it thoroughly but it's equally gorgeous cold on a hot day. This recipe serves four, giving you four meals ready for the week as the soup will last 3–4 days in the fridge. It also freezes well.

COURGETTE, PEA AND MINT SOUP

SERVES 4

1 tsp coconut or olive oil

1 onion, finely diced

3 garlic cloves, very finely chopped

300g frozen peas

3 medium courgettes (about 500g), grated

1 litre vegetable stock

small handful of mint leaves, plus extra to serve

crème fraîche or yoghurt, to serve

salt and black pepper

Heat the oil in a pan and sauté the onion over a medium heat for 3–4 minutes until translucent. Add the garlic and a pinch of salt and pepper and cook for a further minute before adding the peas, grated courgettes and stock. Bring to the boil, then reduce to a simmer and cook for 10 minutes.

Remove from the heat and allow to cool slightly before transferring all the mixture to a blender. Blitz until smooth then add the mint leaves and blitz again. Return to the pan and taste and adjust the seasoning.

Serve with some extra mint leaves, a swirl of crème fraîche or yoghurt and some freshly ground black pepper.

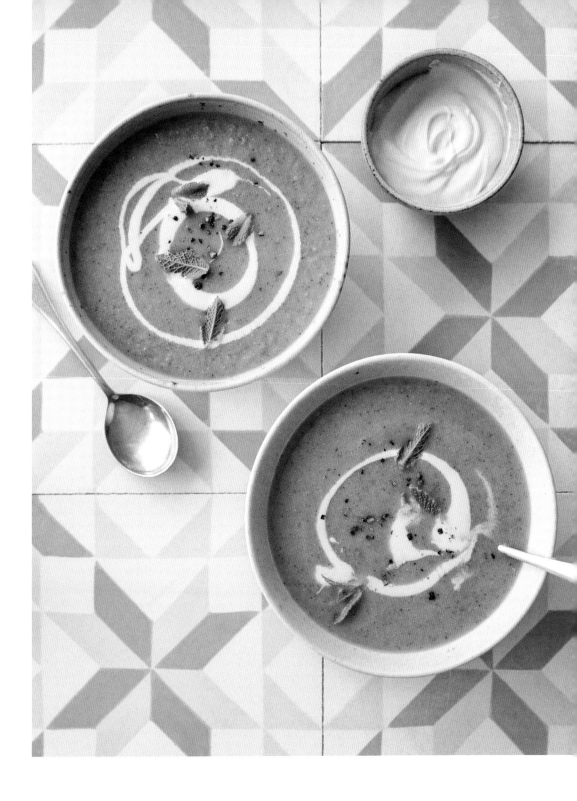

Mackerel is one of the tastiest fish around, plus it contains omega-3 fats, which are essential to our health, with studies even suggesting they reduce our risk of cardiovascular disease. Mackerel also contains vitamin D, 'the sunshine vitamin', so during the winter it's important we get vitamin D from food sources. If you're watching your pennies then mackerel is a great option to have on standby as it's a cheaper option than many other fish!

MACKEREL COBB SALAD

SERVES 2

2 medium eggs

3 slices of bacon, diced

1 small iceberg lettuce, shredded

3 tomatoes, diced

1 ripe avocado, diced

30g blue cheese, crumbled

100g mackerel fillets (smoked or tinned)

For the dressing

3 tbsp olive oil

1 tbsp red wine vinegar

1 tbsp lemon juice

1 tbsp Dijon mustard

1 tbsp Worcestershire sauce

1 garlic clove, very finely chopped

salt and black pepper

Put the eggs into a pan, cover with cold water and place over a high heat. When the water comes to the boil, add a lid, remove from the heat and leave to stand for 10 minutes. (You can boil the eggs any way you like; this is just how I like to do it.) Drain and cool the eggs under cold water. When they are cool enough to handle, peel and cut in half.

Fry the bacon in a small frying pan over a medium-high heat until cooked through and crispy.

Place the lettuce in a serving bowl and top with the tomatoes, avocado, blue cheese and cooked bacon. Finally, flake over the mackerel.

Make up your dressing by whisking together all the ingredients with a pinch of salt and pepper (or shake together in a jar with a tight-fitting lid). Drizzle over the salad and toss to combine – any leftover dressing will keep in a sealed container in the fridge for a few days.

Quinoa is a complete source of protein (see page 30), making it ideal for vegetarian and vegan dishes. Falafel are usually made from just chickpeas, which – unlike quinoa – don't have a complete amino acid profile; this recipe is just as tasty if not better! Try serving this with the Cucumber Tabbouleh and Beetroot Dip and (see pages 163 and 234) or hummus and rice! If you are eating at work, you can pack a wrap separately; come lunchtime just add your salad and falafel, roll it and there you have a tasty falafel wrap!

QUINOA FALAFEL

SERVES 4

170g quinoa

1 x 400g tin chickpeas, drained and rinsed

3 garlic cloves, very finely chopped

1 white onion, finely chopped

2 spring onions, finely chopped

20g parsley, finely chopped

½ tbsp lemon juice

2 tsp ground cumin

1 tsp ground coriander

2 tbsp olive oil, plus extra for brushing

salt and black pepper

Cook the quinoa as per the packet instructions, drain, rinse and allow to cool off a little.

Put the chickpeas into a bowl and mash until broken down but still retaining some texture. Stir through the quinoa, white and spring onions, parsley, lemon juice, cumin, coriander, olive oil and a pinch of salt and pepper.

Transfer all the ingredients to a food processor and pulse until the ingredients start to stick together, but not so much you purée them. You may need to do this in batches.

Using your hands, form the mixture into balls just larger than a golf ball (you should get about 24 falafel). Place on a plate and chill in the fridge for 15 minutes while you preheat the oven to 180°C fan/200°C/400°F/gas mark 6 and line a baking tray with baking paper.

Transfer the falafel to the baking tray and lightly brush the tops with olive oil. Bake in the oven for 35–40 minutes until the outside is crispy and the inside cooked through.

It's important to make sure your diet is varied; after all, variety is the spice of life! I love this paella – it's the perfect option when you want a vegetarian meal that is packed with flavour. It is a great one to share with friends and family – you can add extra protein too, if you wish. Any leftovers will keep in the fridge until the next day but it's best to eat leftovers cold; cooked and reheated rice can contain bacteria that causes food poisoning, particularly if it has not been cooled and stored properly. Cool uneaten rice as quickly as possible, ideally within an hour and keep it in the fridge for no more than a day. Once reheated, always check it is steaming hot before eating, and reheat only once.

VEGGIE PAELLA

SERVES 4

2 tbsp olive oil

1 white onion, finely diced

3 garlic cloves, very finely chopped

1 red and 1 green pepper, deseeded and thinly sliced

200g mushrooms, sliced

1 tbsp smoked paprika

1 tsp chilli flakes

200g paella rice

4 large tomatoes, diced

pinch of saffron, soaked in 1 tbsp hot stock (optional)

500ml vegetable stock

100g frozen peas

100g green beans, cut into 3cm pieces

20 pitted olives

salt and black pepper

chopped parsley and lemon wedges, to serve

Heat the olive oil in a large pan over a medium heat. Add the onion with a pinch of salt and sweat down for 3–4 minutes.

Add the garlic and cook for a further minute before adding the peppers and mushrooms.

Add the spices, allow them to toast slightly before adding the rice, tomatoes, saffron and soaking liquid, if using, and vegetable stock. Bring to the boil, then cover, reduce the heat and let simmer for 10 minutes.

Remove the lid and add the peas, green beans and olives. Season with salt and pepper and cook until the rice is tender and soft, about another 10 minutes. If the rice isn't cooking and the dish is running dry you may need to top up the pan with more water. Taste and adjust the seasoning.

Serve garnished with parsley and lemon wedges.

A light and refreshing salad, this is great paired with grilled fish. Alternatively, just add a portion of protein by crumbling in about 30g feta cheese and you can make a great lunchtime dish to enjoy at home or at work. It will last for up to 3 days in an airtight container.

CUCUMBER TABBOULEH

SERVES 4

85g bulgur wheat or 65g quinoa

1 cucumber, diced

3 tomatoes, diced

2 spring onions, thinly sliced

65g parsley, finely chopped

15g mint leaves, finely chopped

3 tbsp olive oil

2 tbsp lemon juice

salt and black pepper

Rinse and cook the bulgur wheat or quinoa according to the packet instructions until al dente, about 15 minutes. Drain well and allow to cool completely.

Place the cooled grains into a large bowl and stir through the cucumber, tomatoes, spring onions, parsley and mint.

Mix together the olive oil, lemon juice and some salt and pepper. Pour over the salad and stir until well combined.

I know all too well how easy it is to fall into the trap of buying your lunch on-the-go every single day. If budget isn't an issue then it's not the end of the world, as there are now tons of healthy options to buy. However, it's not ideal when you need to watch your wallet, so let's get organised! For those of you with families, this is also super-useful as you can do your children's lunch boxes and just make extra for yourself. I often keep leftovers from the night before and use them for lunch.

BUILD YOUR LUNCHBOX

CHOOSE YOUR PROTEIN	CHOOSE YOUR VEGETABLES	CHOOSE YOUR FRUIT	CHOOSE YOUR CARBOHYDRATE
Chicken drumsticks with a satay side sauce	Veg sticks (peppers, cucumber, celery, carrot, courgette) with nut butter or hummus	Fruit salad	Rice
Leftover Quinoa-crusted Macaroni Cheese (see page 177)	Roasted vegetables	Piece of fruit with yoghurt	Quinoa
Peanut butter porridge	Rainbow salads	Pomegranate seeds or chopped apple for salad toppings	Wholegrain bread
Cooked turkey slices	Vegetable soup (take in a separate flask)		Pasta
30g cheese (I love feta)	Grated vegetables	Dried fruit such as raisins or chopped apricots to add to grains	Flaxseed Crackers (see page 212)
Fillet of poached or smoked fish (poached salmon is lovely)			**CHOOSE YOUR GOOD FAT**
Leftover meatballs or koftas			
Quinoa Falafel (see page 161)			Olive oil-based dips, such as hummus
Tuna mayonnaise			Avocado
Hard-boiled eggs			Nuts
Three-bean salad			Seeds
Cooked sausages			

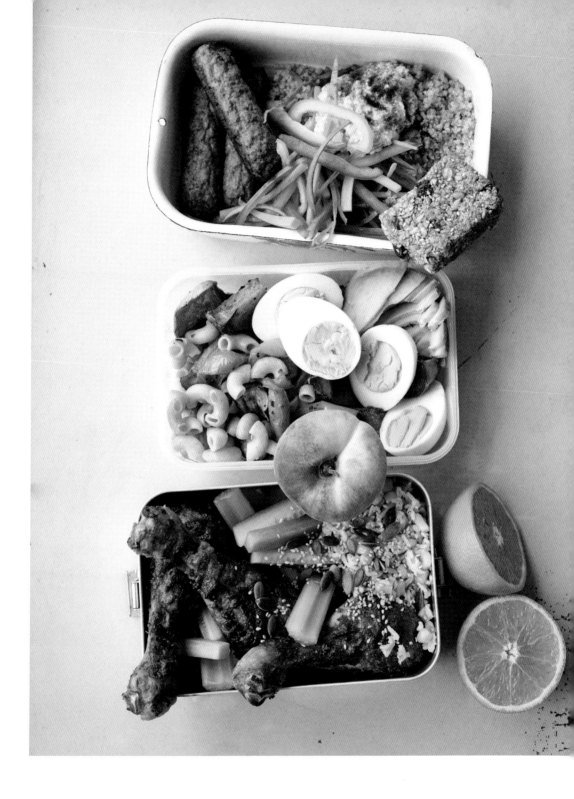

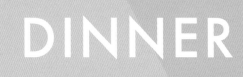

DINNER

At the end of the day there is nothing better than coming home to a scrumptious dinner. There are options here for traditional Friday night favourites, weekend classics and quick and easy dishes for everyone.

I don't often have the will or motivation to slave over a hot stove after a long day in clinic, so you won't find lots of recipes that take ages to prepare or that have a long list of specialist ingredients. These are recipes that are simple, tasty and, most importantly, nourishing!

An English classic. Who says that it can only be enjoyed as a treat?
I wanted to create a version that can be made and enjoyed at home
without a visit to the chippy – and that is much kinder on your waistline
too. You can make it with any white fish fillets, such as cod, hake or
haddock. Just make sure they have been sourced responsibly. There is
also a tofu option for vegetarians and vegans. You can serve it on its
own, but I like to squeeze over some lemon juice and have some of my
home-made Tomato Ketchup and Pea and Mint Purée (see pages 241
and 235) on the side for a bit of colour and some veg.

FISH (OR TOFU) AND CHIPS

SERVES 2

2 large floury potatoes,
such as King Edward

3 tbsp olive oil

salt and black pepper

For the vegan option

1 packet (200g) firm tofu

25g plain or fine
wholemeal flour

20g breadcrumbs

¼ tsp cayenne pepper

1 nori sheet, shredded, or
seaweed flakes (optional)

100ml nut milk or vegan
milk of choice

For the fish option

50g plain or fine
wholemeal flour

1 medium egg beaten

30g breadcrumbs

½ tsp hot or smoked
paprika

2 x 150g white fish fillets

1 tbsp olive oil

First prepare the chips. Preheat the oven to 180°C fan/200°C/
400°F/gas mark 6 while you peel and slice the potatoes into chip
shapes about 1–2cm thick. Toss them in the olive oil and season with
salt and pepper. Tip onto a baking tray and cook for 45 minutes,
or until browned all over and cooked through. Turn them halfway
through cooking so they colour evenly.

If you are making the tofu option, dry the tofu with kitchen paper
and cut lengthways into 3cm slices. Put the flour, breadcrumbs,
cayenne and crumbled nori, if using, into a shallow bowl. Season with
salt and pepper and mix to combine. Put the milk in a second shallow
bowl. Line a baking tray with baking paper. Dip the tofu pieces into the
milk and then into the breadcrumb mixture, making sure the tofu is fully
coated in crumbs. Place on the lined baking tray and bake for
30 minutes (alongside the chips), turning over halfway through.

If you are making the fish option, prepare three shallow bowls –
one with flour, the other with a beaten egg and the third with the
breadcrumbs, paprika and some salt and pepper. Dust the fish in the
flour, then dip into the egg, and then finally send it to the breadcrumb
bowl, making sure you cover all the surfaces with the crumbs. Place
on a lined tray, drizzle with olive oil and bake for 15–18 minutes until
browned on the outside and opaque on the inside. Serve the tofu or
fish and chips with lemon wedges, Ketchup and Pea and Mint Purée.

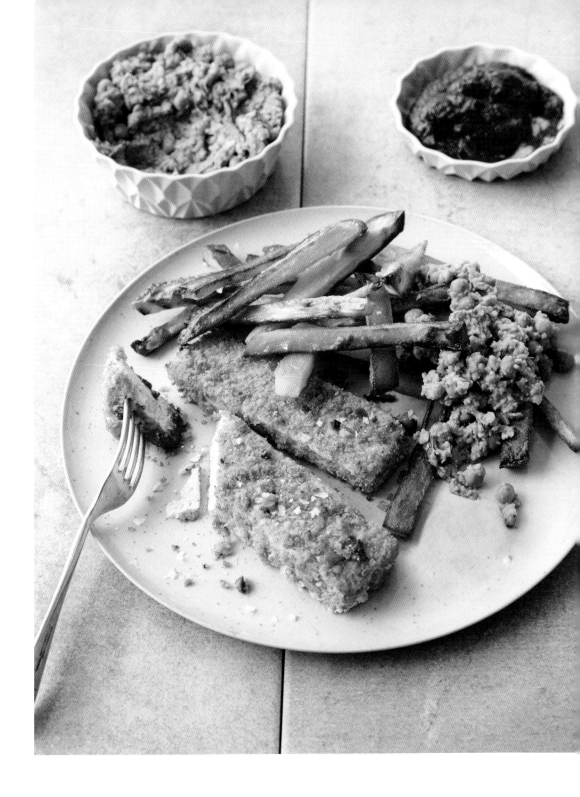

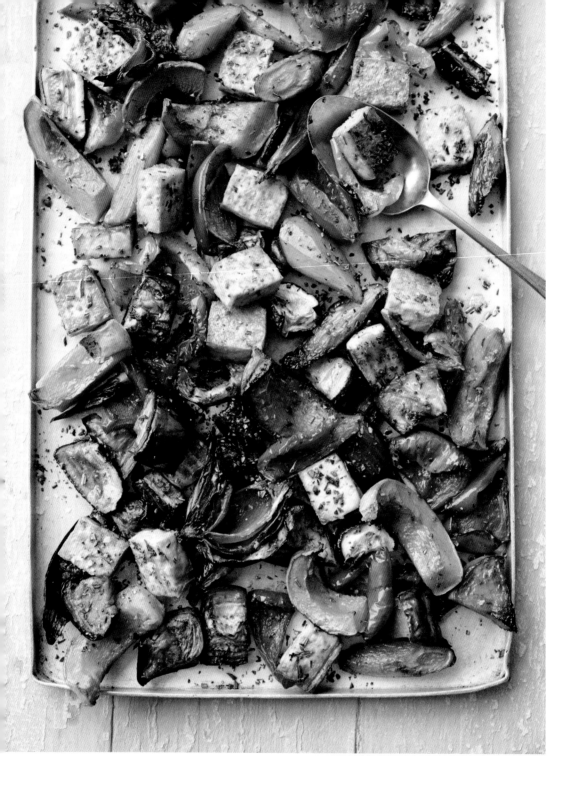

I love tofu and have discovered that it doesn't have to be bland. It's a great source of iron and calcium – both of which are important for a healthy and energised body – so can be enjoyed by meat-eaters as well as vegetarians and vegans. Paired with squash and lots of colourful veg, you can eat a rainbow and reap the benefits at the same time! Try serving this with brown rice, pasta or quinoa.

ROASTED VEGETABLES WITH SQUASH AND TOFU

SERVES 4

2 packets (400g) firm tofu, dried with kitchen paper and cubed

olive oil

1 tbsp lemon juice

4 garlic cloves, very finely chopped

3 sprigs of rosemary, leaves picked and roughly chopped

1 butternut squash, deseeded and cut into 2cm chunks (leave the peel if liked)

1 aubergine, cut into 2cm chunks

2 red onions, peeled and quartered lengthways (with root still attached)

2 courgettes, halved lengthways and cut into 2cm chunks

4 carrots, cut into 2cm chunks

2 peppers, deseeded and cut into 4 pieces

salt and black pepper

Preheat the oven to 180°C fan/200°C/400°F/gas mark 6.

In either a Tupperware, ziplock bag or bowl, combine the tofu with 1 tablespoon of olive oil, the lemon juice, one of the chopped garlic cloves, a pinch of the chopped rosemary and a pinch of salt and pepper. Leave to marinate in the fridge for at least 30 minutes while you roast the veggies.

Place the squash and aubergine on a baking tray and toss with 2 tablespoons of olive oil. Roast for 20 minutes, then add the onions, courgettes, carrots and remaining garlic and rosemary. Season with salt and pepper, toss and return to the oven for a further 10 minutes.

Add the peppers, marinated tofu and any marinade from the bowl and roast for a final 20 minutes.

Fennel is such a versatile ingredient; it's often used raw in salads but can be cooked as well and has a lovely aniseed flavour. Fennel is the perfect accompaniment to chicken and this dish is seriously delicious – I've found it converts even those who don't like fennel! I often serve this with Crunchy Cauliflower Salad (see page 227) or roasted parsnips.

GINGER CHICKEN WITH FENNEL

SERVES 2

For the chicken

juice of 1 lime

½ tbsp soy sauce or tamari

2.5cm piece of fresh ginger, peeled and grated (about 1 tbsp)

1 garlic clove, very finely chopped

2 chicken breasts

For the fennel

1 tbsp olive oil

2 fennel bulbs, ends trimmed, core removed, quartered and thinly sliced

1 red onion, thinly sliced lengthways

1 garlic clove, very finely chopped

2 tbsp vegetable stock

1 tbsp lemon juice

salt and black pepper

In a medium bowl mix together the lime juice, soy sauce or tamari, grated ginger and garlic. Add the chicken to the bowl and coat it with the marinade. Cover and leave in the fridge for 10–30 minutes to marinate.

Meanwhile, preheat the oven to 180°C fan/200°C/400°F/gas mark 6.

Place the marinated chicken on a baking tray, pour over any spare marinade and bake for 25–30 minutes until the chicken is browned. To check if the chicken is cooked through, slice into the thickest part and check the juices run clear and that there is no pink meat.

Meanwhile, prepare the fennel. Warm the olive oil in a medium pan. Add the sliced fennel, onion, ¼ teaspoon each of salt and pepper and cook over a medium-high heat until they have completely softened, about 15–20 minutes. Add the garlic, cook for about 1 minute then add the stock and stir. Add the lemon juice and then taste and adjust the seasoning.

Serve the chicken with the fennel alongside.

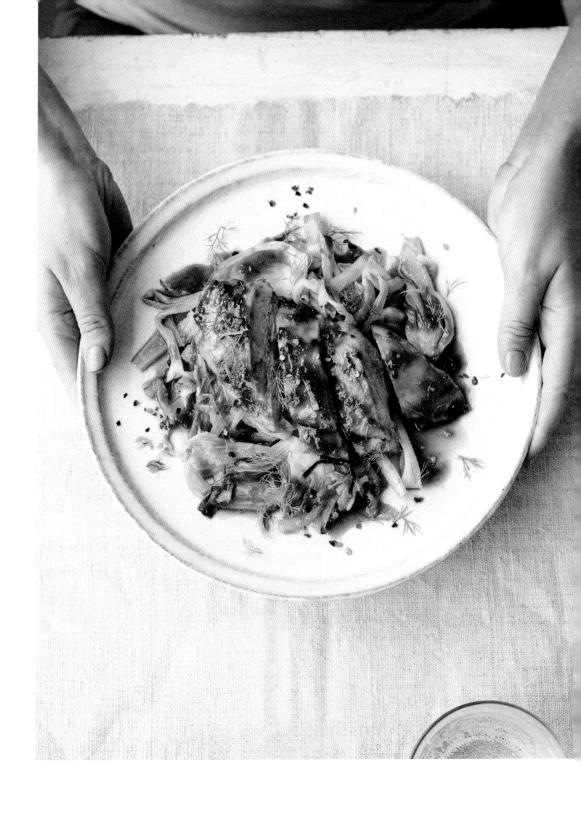

It's important to include a variety of protein sources in your diet, and white fish in particular contains dietary iodine, a crucial element for normal thyroid function. If sea bass isn't your thing, then give any other white fish a go. I like to serve this with my Crunchy Cauliflower Salad (see page 227).

SEA BASS WITH SALSA VERDE AND RICE

SERVES 2

180g brown rice

2 skin-on sea bass fillets, cleaned

2 tbsp olive oil

salt

2 tbsp Salsa Verde (see page 238), to serve

Cook the rice as per the packet instructions; this can take up to 25 minutes, so make sure you allow enough time.

Score the skin of the sea bass, making 4 or 5 shallow cuts into the flesh at about 1cm intervals. Sprinkle over some salt.

Warm a frying pan big enough to hold both sea bass fillets over a medium-high heat and add the olive oil.

Place the fillets skin side down in the pan; they may curl up so use a fish slice to press them flat in the pan. Turn the heat down a little and cook for 2 minutes, or until the skin is crispy and the flesh begins to turn opaque, then flip over and cook for a final minute until done. It may take a little longer to cook (or less time), depending on the thickness of your pieces of fish.

Serve the pan-fried sea bass with the rice, and salsa verde spooned over.

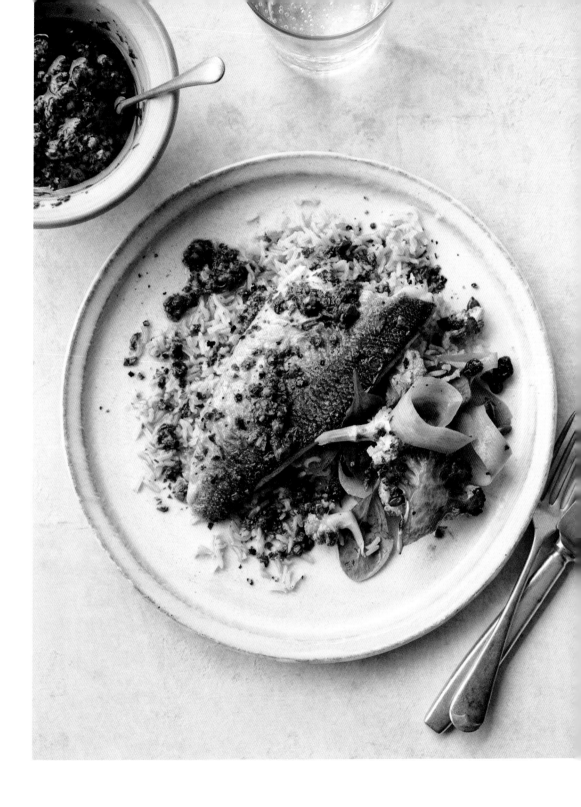

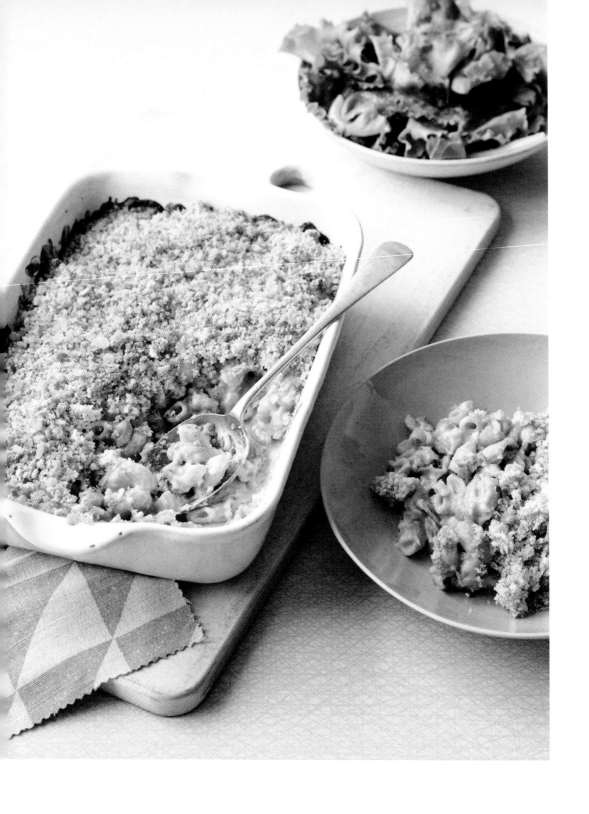

I am sure I am not alone when I say mac 'n' cheese was a childhood favourite. With a few tweaks, this old classic has been reworked to contain more fibre and protein and, if portioned correctly, can be a stand-alone dish or a small side dish.

QUINOA-CRUSTED MACARONI CHEESE

SERVES 4

90g quinoa

30g butter (or use lactose-free butter or olive oil)

30g plain flour (or use gluten-free brown rice flour)

500ml milk of choice

3 garlic cloves, peeled but left whole and lightly crushed

1 tsp Dijon mustard

80g Cheddar, grated (or use a vegan or dairy-free version)

35g Parmesan, grated (or use a vegetarian/vegan or dairy-free version)

pinch of grated nutmeg

300g brown rice pasta (I like elbow macaroni)

90g breadcrumbs (or use gluten-free breadcrumbs)

salt and black pepper

Preheat the oven to 200°C fan/220°C/425°F/gas mark 7.

First cook your quinoa following the instructions on the packet (usually around 15 minutes). If not all the water has been absorbed, drain well and put to one side.

Next make the béchamel sauce. Melt the butter or oil in a medium pan over a low heat, add the flour and stir constantly for about 3 minutes. Slowly add the milk, stirring all the time. Add the garlic and mustard and bring to a simmer. Cook over a low heat, stirring constantly, for about 15 minutes, or until thickened. The sauce is ready when it coats the back of a spoon. Take the pan off the heat, remove the garlic and stir in the Cheddar and half of the Parmesan. Add a grating of nutmeg and salt and pepper to taste.

Meanwhile, cook your pasta following the instructions on the packet. When the pasta is cooked, drain and add it to the béchamel sauce. Stir well and pour into an oven dish.

To make the quinoa crust, combine the cooked quinoa, breadcrumbs, remaining Parmesan cheese and salt and pepper. Scatter this mixture over the mac 'n' cheese and then bake for 20–24 minutes, or until golden and crispy on top.

After returning from a holiday to Africa I was really disappointed that I didn't get to try a local tagine, so I decided to make my own version. You don't need a traditional tagine dish to make this – a good flameproof casserole or ovenproof pan with a lid will be fine. The raisins or dried apricots add a little sweetness to the dish but you can leave them out if you prefer. Turkey is often only thought of as a festive food but it's a really good source of low-fat protein, so you should enjoy it all year round!

TURKEY TAGINE

SERVES 4

2 tbsp olive oil

1 white onion, finely diced

3 garlic cloves, very finely chopped

1 tsp grated fresh ginger

400g turkey breast, cut into 2cm pieces

1 cinnamon stick

2 tsp coriander seeds, toasted and ground

2 tsp cumin seeds, toasted and ground

1 tsp ground turmeric

½ tsp cayenne pepper

1 small butternut squash, peeled, deseeded and cut into large dice

1 aubergine, cut into large dice

1 carrot, cut into small dice

1 x 400g tin chickpeas, drained and rinsed

1 x 400g tin chopped tomatoes

400ml vegetable stock

Preheat the oven to 200°C fan/220°C/425°F/gas mark 7.

In a large flameproof casserole or ovenproof pan (or tagine dish if you have one) heat the olive oil over a medium heat. Add the onion with a pinch of salt and sweat down for 3–4 minutes.

Add the garlic and ginger and sweat for a further minute, then add the turkey and cook for about 5 minutes until it starts to brown. Add all the spices and cook for a minute or so until they become fragrant.

Next add the butternut squash, aubergine, carrot, chickpeas, chopped tomatoes, stock and a tablespoon of lemon juice. Stir to combine and then season to taste.

Bring to the boil, then cover and place in the oven for 1 hour. After 30 minutes, reduce the oven temperature to 150°C fan/ 170°C/325°F/gas mark 3 and give the tagine a good stir.

At the end of the cooking time the meat and vegetables should be incredibly tender. Stir through the raisins or apricots, then taste and adjust the seasoning if necessary, adding more lemon juice if the dish needs a bit of zing. Sprinkle with coriander and serve with brown rice.

1–2 tbsp lemon juice

handful of raisins or
chopped dried apricots

salt and black pepper

handful of coriander,
to garnish

300g cooked brown rice,
to serve

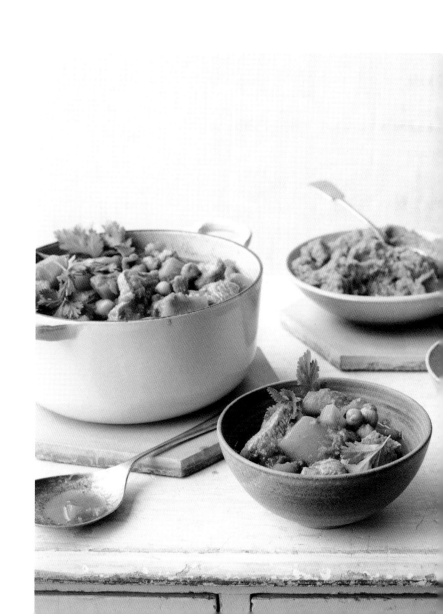

Fish cooked in paper parcels works so well as it keeps the fish moist; these are also incredibly easy to prepare. I just love salmon; it truly is a tasty oily fish bursting with all those healthy omega-3s. This dish is perfect after a long day at work as it doesn't take to long to cook. Serve with Sweet Potato and Garlic Purée (see page 236).

SALMON PARCELS

SERVES 2

2 salmon fillets

1 lemon, zest and juice of ½, the other ½ thinly sliced

1 red pepper, deseeded and thinly sliced

1 green pepper, deseeded and thinly sliced

1 white onion, thinly sliced

6 cherry tomatoes, halved

10 asparagus stalks, woody ends snapped off

1 garlic clove, very finely chopped

2 tsp capers, drained and chopped

1 sprig of rosemary, leaves picked

2 sprigs of thyme

2 tbsp olive oil

salt and black pepper

Preheat the oven to 160°C fan/180°C/350°F/gas mark 4.

Cut two 20 x 25cm rectangles of baking paper (one for each salmon fillet). Place 2 slices of lemon in the middle of each paper then place the salmon on top. Add the peppers, onion, tomatoes and asparagus around the salmon and top with the garlic, capers, lemon zest and juice, rosemary, thyme and a pinch of salt and pepper. Drizzle over the olive oil.

Fold up the two longer edges of one of the rectangles and fold over to form a seal. Twist the ends together to create an enclosed parcel. Repeat to make a second parcel.

Place the parcels on a baking tray and roast for 18 minutes until the fish is cooked through and no longer opaque.

These Middle Eastern-inspired koftas taste delicious – especially when dipped into my Aubergine Hummus (see page 234). Try making them with lamb mince and rosemary for an alternative flavour.

TURKEY AND COURGETTE KOFTAS

SERVES 4

140g courgette, grated

500g turkey thigh mince

handful of mint leaves, finely chopped

handful of parsley leaves, finely chopped

1 garlic clove, very finely chopped

2 tsp ground cumin

pinch of salt and black pepper

1 medium egg, to bind (optional)

olive oil, for brushing

8 long wooden skewers, soaked in water for 30 minutes

Put the grated courgette onto some kitchen paper and squeeze out any excess moisture, then add to a bowl with the turkey mince, herbs, garlic, cumin and seasoning. Mix the ingredients together; if the mixture won't stick together easily, try whisking an egg and adding it in.

Wet your hands and divide the mixture into 8. Form them into sausage shapes and glide them onto the skewers. Transfer to a plate and chill in the fridge for 20 minutes.

Preheat the grill to medium-high and line the grill rack with foil. Brush the koftas with olive oil and grill for 16–18 minutes, turning until browned all over.

Serve these koftas with Cucumber Tabbouleh (see page 163) and Tzatziki (see page 235).

Whether or not you eat meat, it's really important to have vegetarian meals in your diet. This hearty dish is a firm favourite of mine and you can swap the type of bean too if black beans are not your favourite. You could serve this with a jacket potato, with my Parsnip and Avocado Chips (see page 222) or, like here, with cooked brown rice, fresh chilli (or jalapeños), avocado and lime wedges. Delicious!

BLACK BEAN AND MUSHROOM CHILLI

SERVES 4

2 tbsp olive oil

2 white onions, finely diced

4 garlic cloves, finely chopped

250g chestnut mushrooms, thinly sliced

50g button mushrooms, thinly sliced

2 tsp smoked paprika

2 tsp chilli flakes (to taste)

1 tsp ground cumin

1 tsp ground coriander

¼ tsp cayenne pepper

1 carrot, grated

2 x 400g tins black beans, drained and rinsed

1 x 400g tin chopped tomatoes

200ml vegetable stock

juice of 1 lime

handful of coriander

salt and black pepper

In a large pan or frying pan with a lid, warm the olive oil over a medium heat. Add the onions with a pinch of salt and sauté until softened, about 3–4 minutes. Add the garlic and cook for a further minute before adding the mushrooms. Increase the heat a little and cook the mushrooms for 5–10 minutes until they have browned.

Now add all the spices, allowing them to toast and coat all the ingredients. Then add the grated carrot, beans, tomatoes and the stock. Bring to the boil then reduce to a simmer, cover and cook over a low heat for 30–60 minutes, stirring from time to time (a longer cooking time is best for a richer flavour). Remove the lid for the last 5 minutes of cooking to allow some of the excess liquid to evaporate and for the chilli to thicken.

Add the lime juice and season to taste. Serve with brown rice and top with sliced chillies, diced avocado and lime wedges. Roughly tear over the coriander.

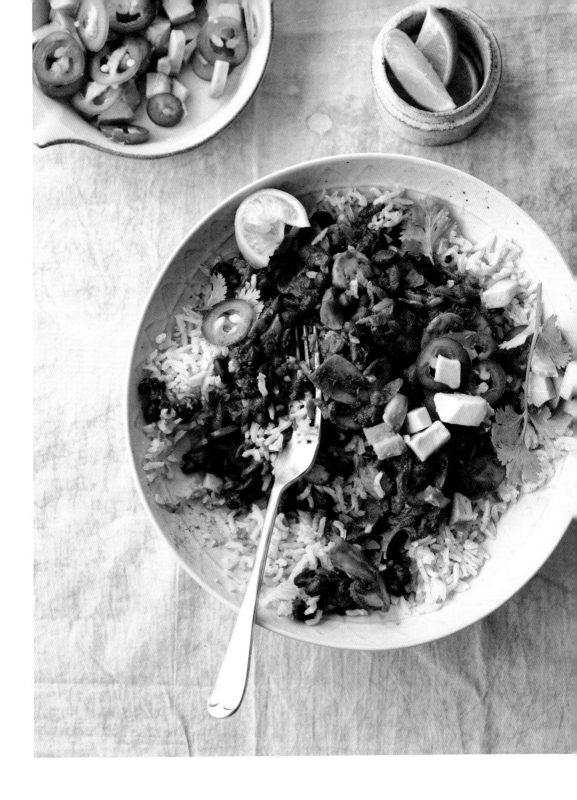

I never used to think I had the time to make soups; now I find there is honestly nothing better. This soup is perfectly balanced and feels like a dish you'd order out! If you don't want to make it with beef you can use turkey mince or add tofu chunks to the broth.

BEEF AND BUCKWHEAT NOODLE SOUP

SERVES 2

For the meatballs

250g beef mince

1 shallot, very finely chopped

1 garlic clove, very finely chopped

1 spring onion, thinly sliced

5cm piece of fresh ginger, peeled and very finely chopped or grated

¼ tsp chilli flakes

pinch of salt and black pepper

1 tsp cornflour (optional)

1 tbsp olive oil

For the broth

1 litre stock

4 garlic cloves, very finely chopped

4 spring onions, thinly sliced

First make the meatballs. Put all the ingredients, except the olive oil, into a bowl and squidge them all together, making sure the aromatics are well distributed. Roll the mixture into 8 large-ish balls, then chill in the fridge until ready to use. (If you are having difficulty getting them to gel together, the cornflour should help.)

Next make the broth. Add the stock to a large pan and bring to the boil. Add the garlic, spring onions, lemongrass, ginger, fish sauce, soy sauce and star anise. Reduce the heat to a simmer and cook for 10 minutes to allow the flavours to infuse.

Meanwhile, heat the olive oil in a frying pan and fry the meatballs for around 8 minutes until they are golden brown all over and cooked through. Turn them frequently.

At the same time put a small pan of water on to boil and cook your noodles following the instructions on the packet (they usually cook in 5–6 minutes). Drain and rinse under cold water.

After the stock has been simmering for 10 minutes, remove the lemongrass and star anise then add the broccoli and cook for a further 5 minutes. When everything else is ready add the spinach and pak choi to the broth; they should wilt down very quickly.

1 lemongrass stalk, bashed (give it a good whack on your counter)

5cm piece of fresh ginger, peeled and very finely chopped or grated

1 tbsp fish sauce

1 tbsp soy sauce

1 star anise

90g buckwheat noodles

60g broccoli florets

60g spinach leaves

90g pak choi

To serve

juice of 1–2 limes

handful of coriander, roughly chopped

handful of mint leaves, roughly chopped

2 spring onions, thinly sliced

1 tsp sesame seeds

You should now be ready to serve. Split the noodles between two serving bowls, add your meatballs and pour the broth over. Add plenty of lime juice and then garnish with coriander, mint, spring onions and sesame seeds.

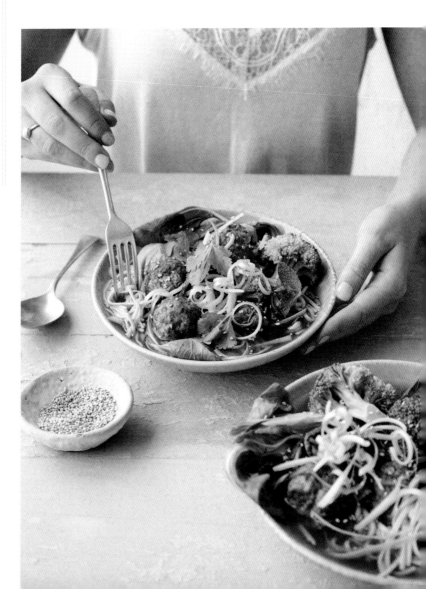

This is a firm favourite of mine – as a child I always looked forward to a shepherd's pie. Nowadays I have my own take on it, using vibrant sweet potatoes to add a naturally sweeter finish. You can easily make this vegetarian or vegan using quorn mince, and remember that it freezes well too. It's also a good one to feed a crowd – just double the quantities.

RE-NOURISH SHEPHERD'S PIE

SERVES 4

For the topping

600g sweet potatoes, peeled and chopped into 2cm chunks

1 tbsp butter (or use coconut oil)

1 garlic clove, thinly sliced

1 tsp dried rosemary

grated zest of 1 lemon

1 tbsp olive oil

salt and black pepper

For the base

1 tbsp olive oil

1 onion, finely chopped

1 carrot, thinly sliced

2 garlic cloves, very finely chopped

few sprigs of thyme, leaves picked

500g beef or quorn mince

175g mushrooms, roughly chopped

6 small sun-dried tomatoes

Put the sweet potatoes into a large pan of cold water and place over a high heat. Bring to the boil, then simmer for 10–15 minutes, or until fork tender.

Drain the potatoes, making sure they are as dry as possible, before returning them to the same pan. Add the butter or coconut oil and season with a pinch of salt and pepper. Mash until smooth, then set aside.

Meanwhile start preparing the base. Add the olive oil to a large pan and sauté the onion and carrot over a medium heat for 3–4 minutes, then add the garlic and thyme. Now add the mince and cook for 5–10 minutes, or until browned all over.

Add the mushrooms, sun-dried tomatoes and oil from the jar. Cook for a further 2–3 minutes, then add the stock, lentils, balsamic vinegar and red wine, if using. Bring to the boil, then reduce to a simmer and cook for another 15–20 minutes until the sauce is thickened and reduced. Meanwhile, preheat the oven to 180°C fan/200°C/400°F/gas mark 6.

Stir in the parsley, season to taste and transfer the mixture to a baking dish, about 25 x 30cm. Spread the mash over the top, scuffing it up with the back of a spoon or a fork. Sprinkle over the garlic slices, rosemary, lemon zest and olive oil. Transfer to the oven for 10 minutes, or until piping hot, and finish off under the grill for a crispy golden top. I like to serve this with some grated cheese on top to finish.

from a jar, roughly
chopped, plus 2 tbsp oil
from the jar

50ml vegetable stock

150g cooked puy lentils
(use ready-cooked from a
tin or packet or cook 75g
dried lentils)

1 tbsp balsamic vinegar

50ml red wine (optional)

handful of parsley,
chopped

salt and black pepper

A NOTE ON MIGHTY MINCE

Mince is such a versatile source of protein and if you're not a red meat eater then why not give turkey mince a try or quorn mince for vegetarians or vegans. Get creative, you can add anything you like and turn it into a completely different item of food. This shepherd's pie, the koftas on page 181 and the meatballs for the soup on page 184 can all be frozen so why not double up?!

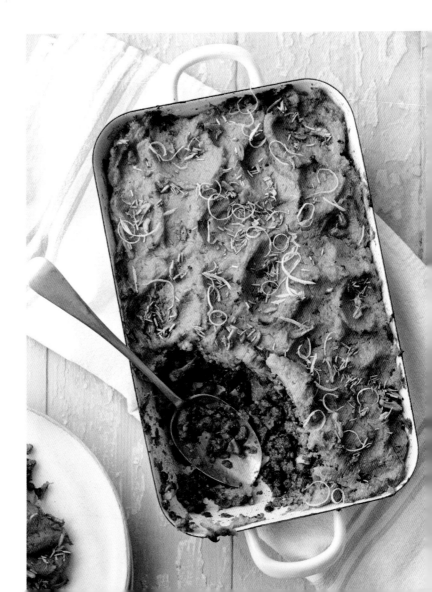

This has become my signature dish at home. When I first moved to London I went to a dinner party with my friends at the Royal Academy of Music, most of whom were international students, so we all tried our own cultural dishes. The Thai students' curry was so amazing I asked for the recipe; consequently this curry became the first recipe I learnt to cook myself. It's so delicious and – best of all – simple to make!

THAI PRAWN CURRY

SERVES 4

1 tbsp coconut oil

2 onions or 4 shallots, finely chopped

1 garlic clove, very finely chopped

1 red pepper, deseeded and thinly sliced

2 green peppers, deseeded and thinly sliced

2 courgettes, thinly sliced

2 tbsp Thai red or green curry paste (check the label for no added sugar)

1 x 400ml tin coconut milk

360g raw or cooked prawns (if frozen, defrost fully before using)

juice of 1 lime

bunch of coriander, roughly chopped

Heat the oil in a wok or large pan. Add the onions or shallots and sauté for 3–5 minutes until soft and translucent. Add the garlic along with the peppers and courgettes and cook for another 5 minutes.

Stir in the curry paste and cook for 1 minute, stirring all the time, then add the coconut milk. Bring to the boil, then reduce the heat to a simmer.

If you are using raw prawns, add them now and simmer for 10 minutes until they are pink and cooked through. Keep stirring the curry to stop it sticking and keep the prawns submerged in the liquid. If you are using cooked prawns, simmer the vegetables for just 5 minutes, then add the cooked prawns and simmer for 1 minute until heated through.

Taste and add a little more curry paste or salt if you think it needs it. Add the lime juice and half the coriander and then serve with your choice of Thai jasmine, basmati or brown rice (or you could even try cauliflower rice for a lighter option). Scatter over the remaining coriander.

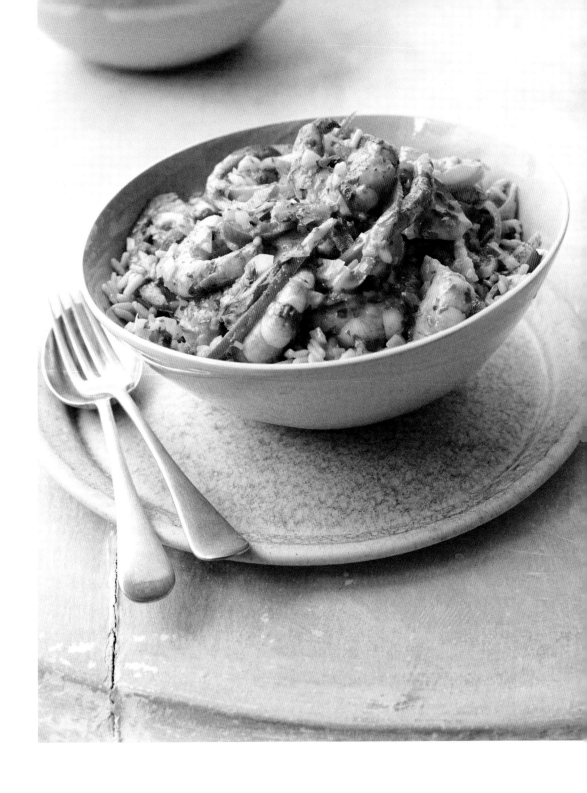

SWEET TREATS

I am not the sort of nutritionist who believes in zero sugar forever and always – I honestly love dessert as much as the next person. It's all about moderation and of course adaptation. I don't advise having dessert every day – perhaps once or twice a week – but it all depends upon your lifestyle and goals.

I have included here some healthier takes on my favourite desserts. These will still give you nourishment but if weight loss is on your agenda they should be seen as a treat, not an everyday occurrence. That being said, you will find that some of these recipes are super-virtuous while others are a tad more indulgent, so there really is something for everyone!

I would always go for a crumble over a pie; it is one of my all-time favourites. I've tweaked the recipe and made a flourless topping with oats and almonds to give an extra protein punch. Cinnamon and apple work well together but if you have other firm fruit that needs using up, such as peaches or plums, you can always use those instead. Serve with a scoop of ice cream or yoghurt.

APPLE CRUMBLE

SERVES 4–6

For the apple base

600g eating apples (e.g. Braeburn or Gala), peeled, cored and cut into chunks

60g berries of your choice

juice of 1 orange

2 tbsp honey

1 tsp ground cinnamon

For the crumble topping

100g rolled oats

40g ground almonds

2 tsp ground cinnamon

4 tbsp butter or coconut oil (cold)

2 tbsp honey

Preheat the oven to 180°C fan/200°C/400°F/gas mark 6.

Put the apples, berries, orange juice, honey and cinnamon into a baking dish and pour over 3 tablespoons of water. Stir gently to combine.

To make the topping, put half the oats into a food processor and blitz to a flour. Tip into a bowl and stir in the rest of the oats, the ground almonds and cinnamon. Rub the butter (or solid coconut oil) into the mixture with your fingertips, then mix in the honey too.

Spread the crumble on top of the apple base and bake in the oven for 30–40 minutes, or until the crumble is golden brown on top.

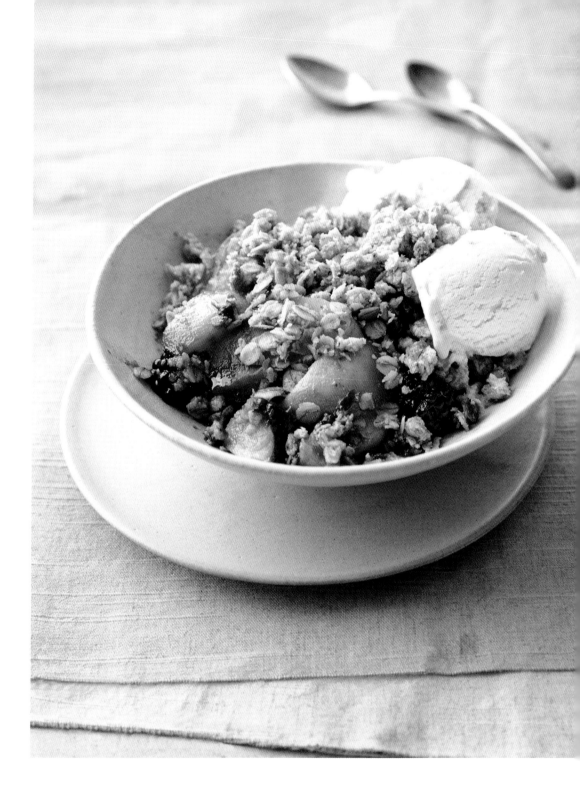

If you need a healthy dish to impress, try this tart. Dried apricots contain fibre, vitamin A (from the beta-carotene) and catechins (flavonoid phytonutrients) – I prefer the organic, brown unsulphured variety. Pecans are packed with heart-healthy fats, meaning you can enjoy a slice knowing you are still providing your body with nourishment.

PECAN AND APRICOT TART

SERVES 10–12

For the pastry

160g finely milled plain wholemeal flour

¼ tsp sea salt

½ tsp sugar or honey

½ tsp grated orange zest

100g chilled and solid coconut oil, plus extra for greasing

4–6 tbsp ice-cold water

For the filling

3 medium eggs

2 tbsp coconut oil, melted

60g honey

1 tbsp milk of choice

1 tsp vanilla extract

1 tsp ground cinnamon

½ tsp ground nutmeg

½ tsp grated orange zest

pinch of salt

220g pecans

First make the pastry: put the flour, salt, sugar, if using, and orange zest in a food processor and pulse to combine. Add the solid coconut oil in chunks, and pulse again until the mixture becomes crumbly.

Add the honey, if using, to the processor, followed by the cold water, a tablespoon at a time. Pulse and add more water until a dry dough comes together. Remove from the processor, shape the dough into a disc, wrap in cling film and chill in the fridge for 20 minutes. Meanwhile, preheat the oven to 180°C fan/200°C/400°F/gas mark 6 and lightly grease a 20cm loose-bottomed tart tin. (I used a fluted tart tin but you don't have to.)

Remove the chilled pastry from the fridge, unwrap and place on a floured surface. Take a floured rolling pin and roll out the pastry to a roughly 30cm circle. Carefully transfer the pastry to the prepared tin, gently pressing the pastry into the bottom and sides. Trim the edges but leave a slight overlap.

Line the pastry with baking paper, add baking beans (I use dried borlotti beans) and bake for 15 minutes until the bottom of the tart is no longer raw and it is just starting to brown. Remove from the oven and remove the paper and baking beans. Return the tart case to the oven for a further 5 minutes. Remove from the oven and increase the oven temperature by 20°C.

3 tbsp finely milled plain
wholemeal flour

150g dried apricots,
soaked in hot water for
5 minutes, drained and
finely chopped

While the pastry is blind baking, make your filling. Place the eggs,
melted coconut oil, honey, milk, vanilla, cinnamon, nutmeg, orange
zest and salt in a bowl and whisk together – by hand or with an electric
whisk – until well combined and a little frothy. Finely chop 120g of the
pecans and add to the bowl with the flour; fold in by hand.

Scatter the apricots over the pastry base, then pour over the filling.
Arrange the remaining whole pecans on top of the filling in a pretty
pattern. Bake in the oven for 10 minutes, then turn down the temperature
by 20°C and cook for another 15–20 minutes until the eggy top is set
and browned.

Remove from the oven and allow to cool before slicing. Serve with a
dollop of Greek yoghurt or some tasty ice cream.

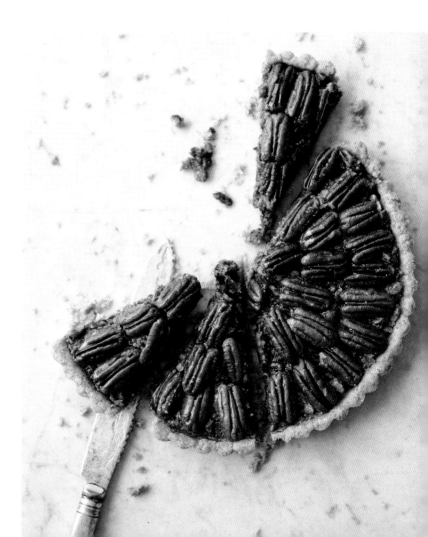

I often prepare this dessert in advance to enjoy later that evening or the following day (it keeps well in the fridge). Pears are best when in season (see page 110) and a pear's window of optimum ripeness is smaller than that of apples. Store at room temperature to accelerate ripening and refrigerate ripe pears or those you won't be using for a few days. This dish is best made with slightly firm pears.

POACHED PEAR AND FIG

SERVES 4

pared zest and juice
of 1 orange

1 tbsp honey (optional)

1 vanilla pod, split
lengthways (or use 1 tsp
vanilla extract)

1 cinnamon stick

1 star anise

1 whole clove

2 firm pears, peeled,
quartered and cored

4 figs, halved and
hard tips removed

Greek yoghurt, coconut
yoghurt or cream, to serve

Put 400ml water into a pan large enough to hold the pears. Add the orange zest and juice, honey, if using, and spices. Bring to the boil, then reduce the heat to a simmer.

Add the pears and figs and simmer for around 25 minutes, until a knife glides easily into the pear and the figs are soft. Remove the fruit and transfer to a bowl.

If you'd like you can reduce the remaining liquid to form a syrup. Return the pan to the heat, increase to high and let it bubble away for about 5 minutes until thick and syrupy.

Pour the syrup back over the strained fruit then chill in the fridge until ready to serve.

Desserts can often enhance your daily diet; if you haven't had your fruit for the day then finishing it with a gorgeous baked apple is a good idea – apples are a good source of both fibre and vitamin C. They also contain polyphenols, which can have numerous health benefits.

BAKED CINNAMON APPLE WITH RAISINS

SERVES 4

4 firm and sweet eating apples (e.g. Braeburn or Gala)

50g raisins

½ tbsp olive oil

1 tsp ground cinnamon

¼ tsp ground nutmeg

Preheat the oven to 180°C fan/200°C/400°F/gas mark 6 and line a baking tray with baking paper.

Cut apples in half, through the stem, and remove the core and pips using a spoon, making enough room for the filling (a sharp spoon like a melon baller makes this a breeze). Place on the lined baking tray.

Mix together the remaining ingredients and then spoon the mixture into the well of each apple.

Bake in the oven for 25–30 minutes, until the apple flesh has softened and browned on top. Serve with a nice big dollop of Greek yoghurt.

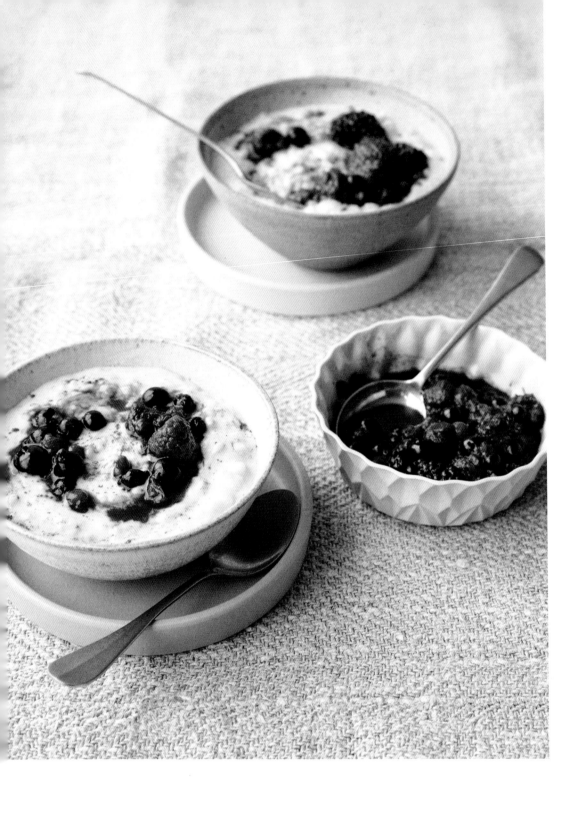

This has become a firm favourite in my family. You can choose your preferred milk and some clients even swap the rice for quinoa, for an added protein boost. Berries are high in antioxidants such as anthocyanins, which may protect cells from free radical damage; they are also high in fibre and low in calories, so tuck in!

BERRY RICE PUDDING

SERVES 2

400ml milk (or use a plant-based or dairy-free alternative)

100g pudding rice

10g honey

2 tsp vanilla extract

½ tsp ground cinnamon

For the berries

200g mixed berries (fresh or frozen)

½ tsp vanilla extract

Put the milk into a small pan and bring to the boil, then reduce to a simmer. Add the rice, honey, vanilla and cinnamon, stir well, then cover and cook over a low-medium heat for 25–30 minutes, making sure you stir frequently to prevent it from sticking to the pan.

Meanwhile, put the berries, 2 tablespoons of water and vanilla into another small pan and warm over a medium heat for 2 minutes, then cover the pan and cook for a further 2 minutes, by which point the fruit should be starting to soften, and the natural juices should have been released. Remove the lid, turn up the heat to medium-high and cook for a further 2 minutes to bubble away some of the juices.

Serve the pudding in small dessert bowls with the warm berries on top.

I've used buckwheat flour and chocolate protein powder but you can use any flour you like, and vanilla protein powder would work just as well. These pancakes are a healthy dessert item and can also act as a great breakfast option – they are high in protein and will leave you full and satisfied.

CHOCOLATE PROTEIN PANCAKES

SERVES 2

1 small banana

1 medium egg (omit for vegan pancakes, as long as you include the banana)

140ml milk of choice

1 tsp honey (optional)

20g chocolate protein powder

20g buckwheat flour

1 tbsp 100% unsweetened cocoa powder or raw cacao powder

1 tsp baking powder

coconut or olive oil, for frying

To serve

yoghurt, berries, nut butter, maple syrup, honey, chopped nuts or Chocolate Sauce (see page 242)

Put the banana into a bowl and mash with a fork. Whisk in the egg, milk and honey, if using. Then add all the dry ingredients and whisk again. (Alternatively you can just whizz everything together in a blender.)

Warm a large frying pan over a medium heat, add 1 tablespoon of oil and swirl it around the pan. Dollop in around 1 heaped tablespoon of the batter mixture to make an American-style thicker pancake, then continue to add 2 or 3 to the pan (don't overcrowd the pan as it makes them difficult to flip). Cook for 2–3 minutes each side, only flipping when the underside is browned and has formed a light crust. Remove from the pan when done on both sides and continue with the rest of the batter.

Plate the pancakes up in a stack and serve with your favourite toppings.

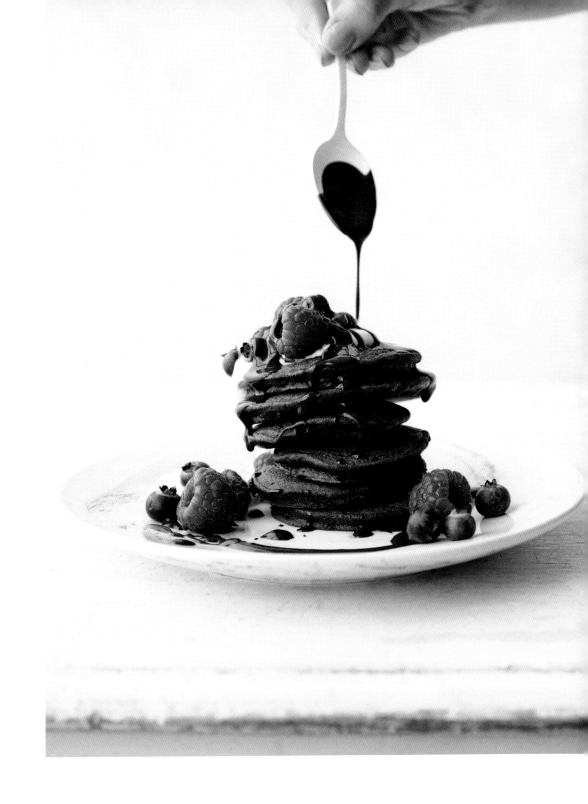

This is a completely no-fuss, simple and waistline-friendly dessert that is perfect when you just need a chocolate fix! You can use coconut yoghurt to make this suitable for vegans but I tend to use Greek yoghurt as it's thicker and creamier. This bowl will keep you full and satisfied, and you will be enriching your body with phytonutrients, protein, healthy fats and calcium.

CACAO YOGHURT BOWL

SERVES 1

125ml milk of choice

100g yoghurt of choice

1 banana or ½ avocado (you may need additional sweetener if using avocado)

2 tbsp good-quality cocoa powder or raw cacao powder

1 tbsp coconut flour, to thicken

1–2 tsp honey, to taste

Topping ideas

50g berries (I love frozen raspberries)

15g dried mulberries or cranberries

1 tbsp coconut flakes

Put the milk, yoghurt, banana or avocado, cocoa, coconut flour and honey into a blender and blitz until smooth. Taste and adjust if necessary: you may need more honey if you've used avocado instead of banana. You can also add more cocoa powder if you want more of a chocolate hit.

Pour into a bowl and top with berries, dried fruit or coconut flakes.

If you have a sweet tooth then having a nice mug of hot chocolate can be the perfect way to curb those chocolate cravings. There is considerable evidence that cocoa can provide powerful health benefits; however, this doesn't mean people should go all out and eat masses of chocolate every day. Try this hot drink to get some benefit without damaging your waistline. Raw cacao is also suggested to have more health benefits than cocoa powder. (See page 88 for a photograph.)

HOT CHOCCY

SERVES 1

1 tbsp good-quality cocoa powder or raw cacao powder

1 tsp honey

1 tsp nut butter (optional, for home-made see page 243)

250ml almond milk (or any milk of choice)

½ tsp ground cinnamon

In a small pan, make a smooth paste with the cocoa powder, honey, nut butter, if using, and a couple of tablespoons of the milk.

Place over a medium heat and, using a balloon whisk, whisk in the rest of the milk. Keep whisking to ensure bits don't get stuck to the bottom of the pan, while the cocoa heats up to the perfect drinking temperature (don't allow the mixture to boil).

Whisk in the cinnamon, pour into a mug and enjoy!

SNACKS

Snacking is a really smart and effective way to make sure you're not absolutely ravenous come dinnertime. Allowing yourself to get overly hungry will only encourage overeating. The snack choice you make is crucial as to whether it will keep you full and maintain any healthy eating regime.

I am frequently asked what items make new and exciting snacks. If you're often on the go, I tend to encourage foods with fibre and protein to ensure you keep a steady blood sugar balance (see page 24). I have created a variety of options, which can be eaten at home or taken with you in your bag.

These are great for afternoon snacks, and go well with all the dips in the following chapter. They contain healthy fats and protein, helping us feel satisfied for longer, plus you also have the option of using wholemeal flour for some additional fibre and nutrients.

MINI MEXICAN MUFFINS

SERVES 12

4 tbsp olive oil

1 red pepper, deseeded and diced into small pieces

1 tbsp pumpkin seeds, plus extra for the topping

1 tbsp sunflower or poppy seeds, plus extra for the topping

200ml milk of choice

1 medium egg

300g self-raising flour (use wholemeal self-raising flour if you can find it)

1 tsp hot or smoked paprika

½ tsp salt

pinch of black pepper

handful of chopped coriander (optional)

20g Cheddar, grated, plus extra for the topping (optional)

butter, to finish (optional)

Preheat the oven to 180°C fan/200°C/400°F/gas mark 6 and line a 12-hole shallow muffin tray with paper cases.

Warm 1 tablespoon of the olive oil in a frying pan over a medium heat and sauté the diced pepper for 3–4 minutes. Add the seeds to the pan and toast for a final minute, stirring often.

Put the milk, remaining olive oil and egg into a bowl and beat together with a fork or small whisk. In a second bowl combine the flour, paprika, salt and pepper and coriander and cheese, if using.

Tip the cooked peppers into the egg mix, stirring to distribute them. Gently fold in the flour mixture, taking care not to overwork the mixture. The batter should be fairly stiff.

Using two spoons as scoops, divide the muffin batter evenly between the paper cases. Sprinkle with a few extra seeds, then bake in the oven for 15–18 minutes until browned on top and a skewer inserted into the middle comes out clean.

If you like, add an optional teaspoon of butter to the top of each warm muffin and sprinkle with a little extra cheese. Transfer to a wire rack and allow them to cool slightly before eating – they are delicious warm but can be eaten cold.

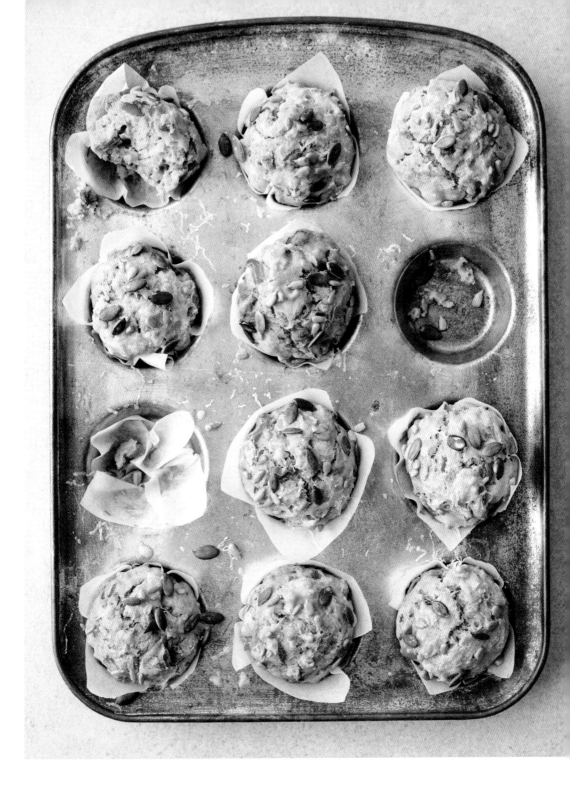

When making a batch of these squares remember that they'll keep for a few days – another option is to freeze them and just take them out of the freezer to defrost in the fridge the night before you want them. These granola squares also make a great pre-workout snack!

GRANOLA SQUARES

MAKES 12–16

4 tbsp nut butter (for home-made see page 243)

4 tbsp honey

2 tbsp coconut oil

150g rolled oats

3 tbsp desiccated coconut

40g raisins

40g chopped almonds

20g sunflower seeds

25g sesame seeds

Preheat the oven to 180°C fan/200°C/400°F/gas mark 6 and line a 20cm square baking tray with baking paper.

Put the nut butter, honey and coconut oil into a small pan over a low heat and warm until it has melted. Stir well.

Meanwhile, put all the rest of the ingredients into a bowl and stir so the ingredients are evenly distributed. Pour the wet ingredients into the bowl and stir until well combined and all of the mixture is coated.

Press into the baking tray and, using a sharp knife, lightly score the top into a grid of 12–16 squares or rectangles; this will make it easier to cut them when baked.

Bake in the oven for 10–15 minutes until browned and firm to the touch. Leave to cool fully before slicing into squares along the lines you pre-scored.

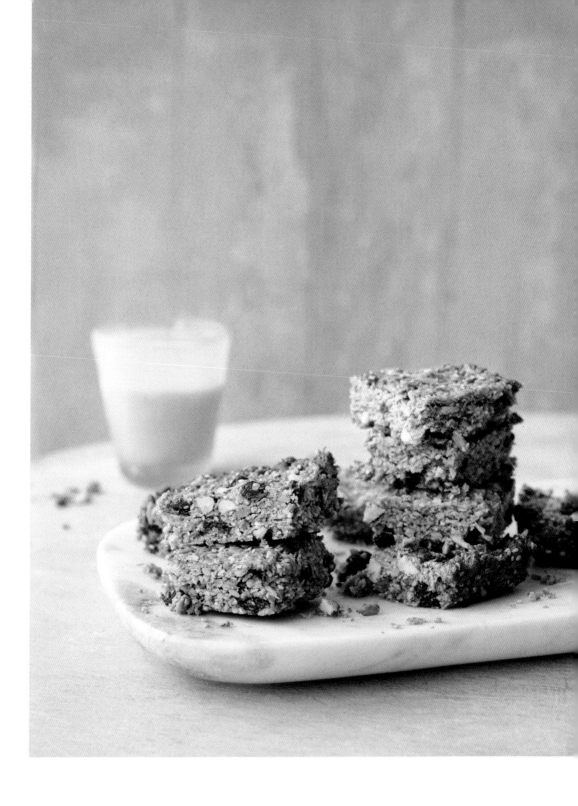

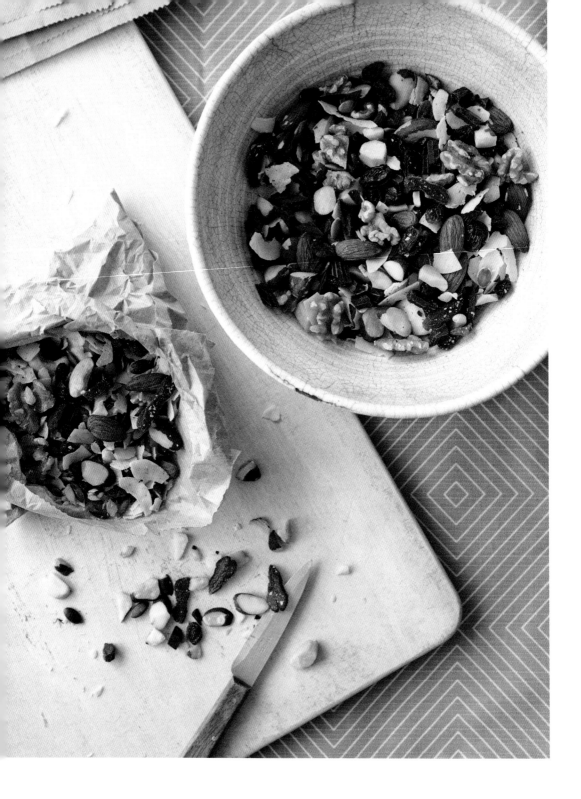

These are perfect for when you're on-the-go and are not too much hassle to prepare. Just pop some into your bag and when you start to feel hungry you can just grab a handful. You can use any combination of nuts and seeds depending on what you like and what you have in your cupboards – just make sure you use unsalted nuts.

TRAIL MIX

MAKES ABOUT 250G (8 X 30G SERVINGS)

30g walnuts

30g almonds

30g cashew nuts

15 brazil nuts, roughly chopped

30g pumpkin seeds

30g sunflower seeds

25g dried coconut flakes

25g raisins

5 dried apricots, diced (I prefer the organic, unsulphured variety)

20g dark chocolate, roughly chopped (optional)

Combine all the ingredients together and store in an airtight container.

Flaxseeds, also known as common flax or linseeds, are small oily seeds that originated in the Middle East thousands of years ago. Lately, they have been gaining popularity as a health food. This is because they contain heart-healthy omega-3, fibre and other unique plant compounds. I love adding them to porridge but you can make your own healthy crackers with them too! They are linked to a number of health benefits, such as improved digestive function and reduced blood pressure.

FLAXSEED CRACKERS AND DIP

SERVES 4

100g ground flaxseeds

2 tbsp whole flaxseeds

2 tsp dried herbs of your choice (rosemary, oregano etc.)

¼ tsp salt

Preheat the oven to 190°C fan/210°C/420°F/gas mark 6 ½ and line a large baking tray with baking paper.

Combine all of the dry ingredients in a bowl. Slowly add 115ml water and stir to bring together into a dough (the dough will be fairly wet).

Spread the mixture out on the baking tray and, using slightly wet fingers, press and smooth it out evenly to around 1–2mm thick. Use a sharp knife to score the dough into a grid to the desired size of your crackers. This will make them easier to break apart later.

Bake in the oven for 30–35 minutes until browned and crisp all over (you may want to rotate the baking tray in your oven halfway through baking for even colouring). Remove from the oven and let them cool fully before breaking up into their individual crackers.

Serve the crackers with any of the dips in the following chapter (see pages 232–5).

A lot of protein balls contain sugar, which to me makes them counterproductive as a snack – but they are so convenient to transport and keep well throughout the day. Hence this tasty sugar-free version!

PROTEIN BALLS

MAKES 8

30g rolled oats or quinoa flakes

1 scoop (30g) chocolate protein powder (sweetened with stevia only)

2 tbsp hemp seeds or ground flaxseeds

2 tbsp almond butter or peanut butter

1 tbsp raw cacao powder or 100% unsweetened cocoa powder

1 tsp ground cinnamon

75ml warm water

Place all of the ingredients in a food processor and blitz until the mixture comes together into a large ball.

If the dough is too wet then add some more protein powder; if it's too dry add a little more water.

Roll in to 8 equal-sized balls and chill in the fridge until ready to eat. They are best kept in the fridge in an airtight container, where they will keep for a week; alternatively they will keep for a month in the freezer.

This is another convenient snack to make in advance and keep in the fridge in an airtight container. Chickpeas are high in protein, making this a low-sugar and tasty fibre-rich snack!

OVEN-ROASTED CHICKPEAS

**MAKES 400G
(8 X 50G SERVINGS)**

1 x 400g tin chickpeas, drained and rinsed

2 tbsp olive oil

1 tsp chilli flakes

1 tsp ground cumin

pinch of smoked paprika

pinch of sea salt

Preheat the oven to 200°C fan/220°C/425°F/gas mark 7 and line a baking tray with baking paper.

Tip the chickpeas into a bowl and toss with the olive oil, chilli flakes, cumin, paprika and salt, making sure all the chickpeas are well coated.

Spread out on the lined baking tray and bake on the middle shelf of the oven for 25–30 minutes, stirring every 10 minutes or so to make sure they brown evenly. They will be golden and crisp when done.

Leave to cool before dividing into snack portions!

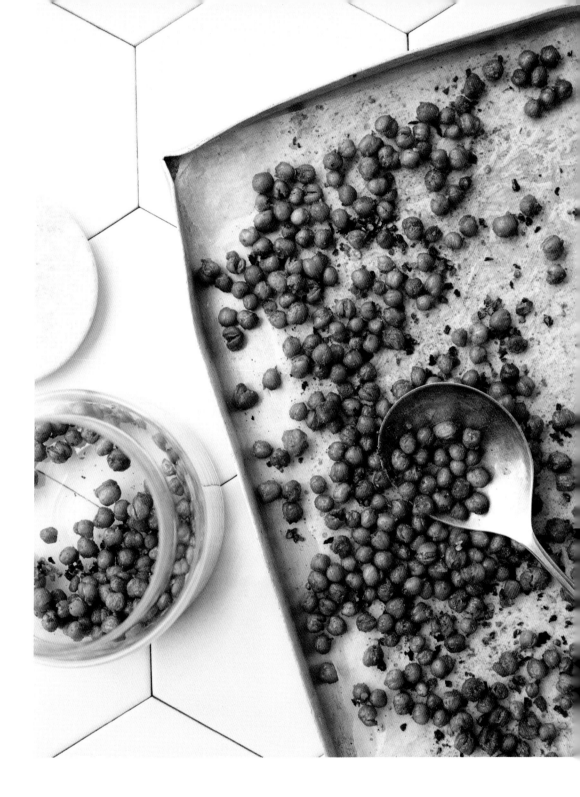

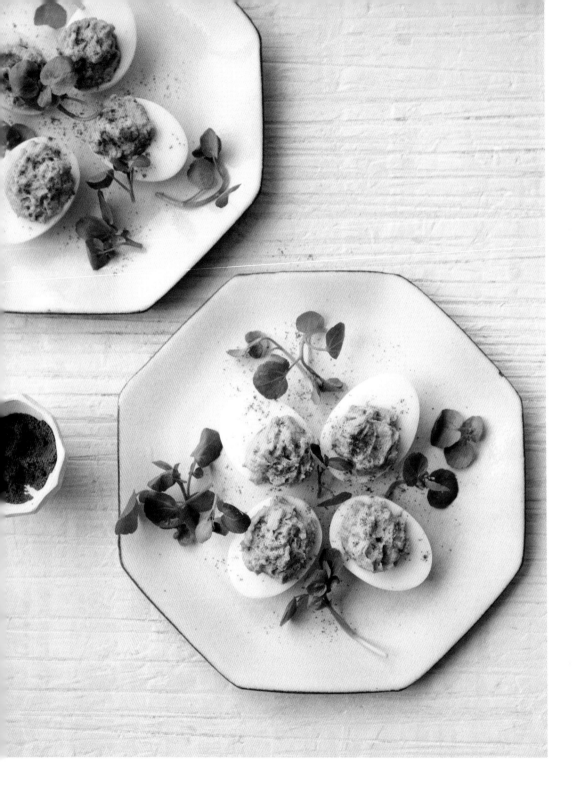

Eggs and avocado are great to snack on as they provide you with healthy fats and protein, keeping you satisfied. But they can be a bit boring on their own, so I decided to combine the two for a spin on this classic. They'd even make a pretty good canapé for a dinner party too! If avocado isn't your thing you can replace it with hummus in this recipe.

SPICY DEVILLED EGGS WITH AVOCADO

SERVES 3

6 medium eggs

1 large ripe avocado, mashed

2 tsp Dijon mustard

¼ tsp smoked paprika

pinch of cayenne pepper, plus extra to serve

pinch of salt and pepper

Put the eggs into a pan, cover with cold water and place over a high heat. When the water comes to the boil, add a lid, remove from the heat and leave to stand for 10 minutes. (You can boil the eggs any way you like; this is just how I like to do it.) Drain and cool the eggs by refreshing under cold water. When they are cool enough to handle, peel the eggs.

Cut the eggs in half lengthways, carefully scoop out the yolks and put them in a bowl. Add the avocado, mustard, paprika, cayenne pepper and salt and pepper and mash until the mixture is smooth and combined.

Fill up the cavity of each egg with the mixture and then chill in the fridge for 20 minutes. Garnish with an extra pinch of cayenne pepper if you like things spicy.

SIDES, DIPS, DRESSINGS AND SPREADS

Side dishes and dips are a fabulous way of adding more variety of colour and flavour to any meal or snack, and the sauces and spreads I've provided here are all simple home-made versions of favourites, without the excess sugar, salt and preservatives you often find.

I find it useful to make lots of these dishes in bulk and keep them for a few days for the week ahead or even freeze some dips in individual containers that I can pull out the night before my friends come over. I'm often asked how to make a meal more interesting in a healthy way or how to jazz up some snack options. The dips go well with lots of the recipes in this book and the snacks and some of the sides can be small dishes in their own right.

This healthy alternative to 'regular' chips would make a fab accompaniment to my Chicken and Roasted Vegetable Skewers (see page 156).

POLENTA CHIPS

SERVES 4

900ml vegetable stock

250g quick-cook polenta

30g Parmesan, finely grated

small handful of parsley, finely chopped

small handful of chives, finely chopped

2 tbsp olive oil

salt and black pepper

Tomato Ketchup (see page 241), to serve

Line a 20 x 30cm baking dish with cling film, leaving the cling film hanging over the edges; set aside.

Put the vegetable stock into a medium pan and bring to the boil. Stirring constantly, add the polenta in a steady stream; continue to stir and cook until the mixture thickens. This should take about 2 minutes.

Stir in the Parmesan, parsley, chives, ½ teaspoon of salt and some black pepper. Allow to cool for a few minutes before pouring into the lined tin. Level the surface and set aside for at least 2 hours, transferring to the fridge when it reaches room temperature. (You can do this up to 2 days in advance – just keep the polenta covered in the fridge until needed.)

When you are ready to cook the chips preheat the oven to 180°C fan/200°C/400°F/gas mark 6.

Lift out the polenta using the cling film overhang and cut the polenta block into slim 'chips'. Carefully toss the pieces with the olive oil and a pinch of salt. Spread out on a large lined baking tray and bake for 25–30 minutes, turning halfway, until golden and crisp. Serve with home-made Tomato Ketchup.

If you're tired of mashed potatoes, polenta is a great alternative; just boil and stir with a wooden spoon. Add the flavourings once it has thickened – traditionally a generous knob of butter and a handful of grated Parmesan, but the key is plenty of seasoning.

CREAMY POLENTA 'MASH'

SERVES 4

½ tsp salt

80g medium-grain yellow polenta

1 tbsp butter

1–2 tbsp cream cheese

salt and black pepper

Bring 470ml water to the boil in a heavy-based pan and add the salt.

Working quickly, stir in the polenta until it is fully incorporated. Lower the heat to a very low simmer, add the butter and allow the polenta to cook gently for 25 minutes until the grains have fully softened. Stir occasionally so it doesn't stick to the bottom of the pan.

Finally, stir in the cream cheese until it has melted into the polenta. Taste and adjust the seasoning – you can also add more cream cheese if you like.

PICK YOUR POLENTA

I love polenta. It is made by grinding corn into flour, giving a rich, yellow, yolk-like colour. It has a slightly sweet flavour, and goes with so many dishes. It's a great cheap store-cupboard staple, not to mention that it contains potassium and vitamin A. Polenta can be served 'wet', like a creamy, thick mashed potato, or allowed to set, sliced and then pan-fried or griddled. Serve it instead of pasta, rice or potatoes or use instead of breadcrumbs to coat chicken or fish when frying, or try dusting onto potatoes before roasting to give them extra crunch. **Traditional polenta** can take up to 50 minutes to cook, depending on the coarseness. Generally it's cooked in boiling water or milk. **Quick-cook or instant polenta** takes just a few minutes to make as it comes part-cooked. Polenta also comes **ready-made in tubes or blocks**, ready to be sliced and reheated.

I put these two together for the natural sweetness from the parsnips and the creamy texture of the avocado. They are a great alternative to regular chips as they will count towards your vegetable intake for the day. Rich in fibre and a multitude of nutrients, these will be a tasty addition to any meal and one that even die hard chip fans will enjoy! Where regular chips are deep-fried, these are simply baked in the oven. I love to serve these with the Pea and Mint Purée on page 235.

PARSNIP AND AVOCADO CHIPS

SERVES 4

For the parsnip chips

450g parsnips, peeled

2 tbsp olive oil, plus extra for greasing

salt and black pepper

For the avocado chips

2 avocados (ripe but still firm), halved, stoned and peeled

50g ground almonds

235ml milk of choice

50g breadcrumbs

salt and black pepper

Preheat the oven to 180°C fan/200°C/400°F/gas mark 6 and lightly grease 2 baking trays with olive oil.

Cut the parsnips into chip shapes, toss with the olive oil and a pinch of salt and pepper in a bowl. Spread out in a single layer on a baking tray, making sure they aren't too crowded.

Cut the avocados into chip shapes slices and prepare three bowls: one with the ground almonds and a pinch of salt and pepper, one with the milk and another with the breadcrumbs. First dip the avocado slices into the almonds, making sure all surfaces are well coated, then dip in the milk, and then into the breadcrumbs, again making sure all the surfaces are well coated. Spread the avocado slices out on the second baking tray.

Bake the parsnips and avocados in the oven for 30 minutes, checking, turning over and rotating the tray halfway cooking to ensure they cook evenly. They will both be done when crispy and brown. Serve hot.

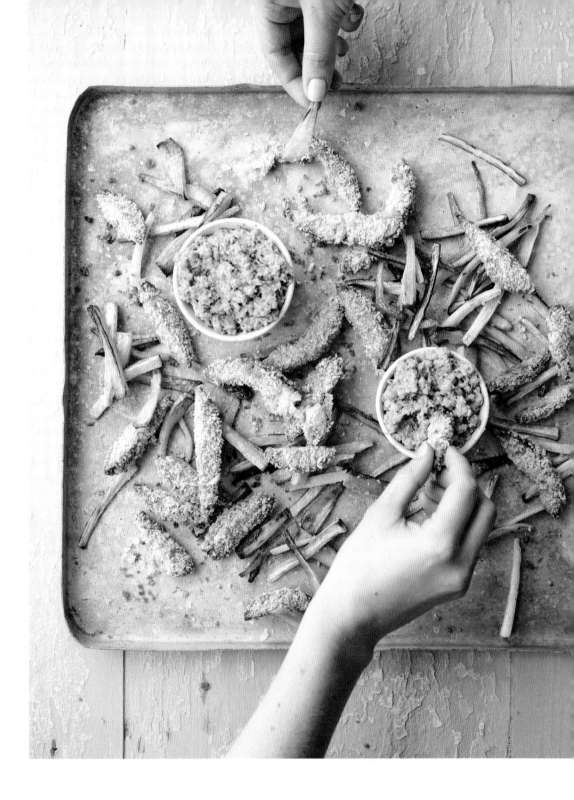

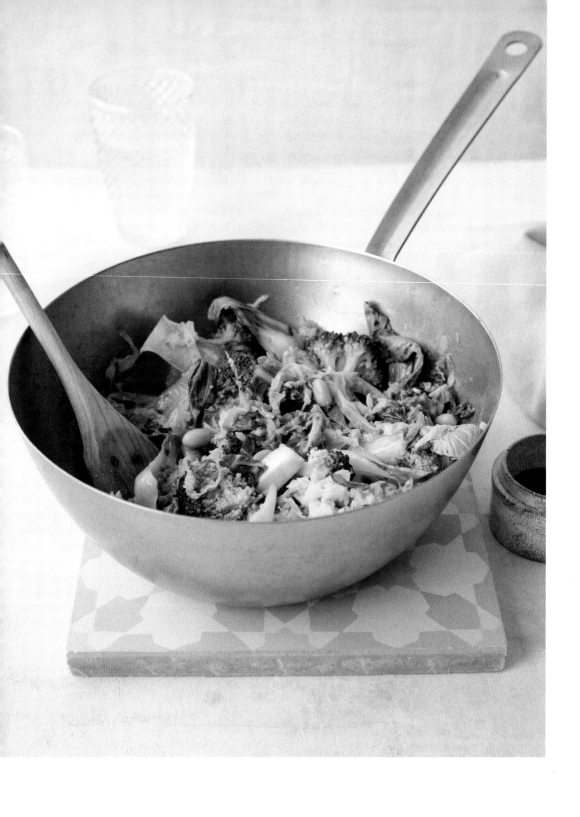

We all need to increase the variety of vegetables in our diet but keeping them interesting and palatable isn't always easy. Miso is a favourite in Asian cuisine, produced by fermenting soybeans, and contains beneficial bacteria for our gut health (see page 46 for more on gut-healthy foods). These greens would go perfectly with a scrumptious salmon fillet or some tempeh. I've used cabbage, broccoli and pak choi but you could swap in any greens that you have in the fridge.

MISO GREENS

SERVES 3–4

90ml warm water

1 tbsp white or brown miso

1 tbsp soy sauce

1 tbsp coconut oil

1 garlic clove, very finely chopped

thumb-sized piece of ginger, finely chopped (about 2 tsp)

½ red chilli, deseeded and very finely chopped

½ medium cabbage (such as savoy), cored and thinly sliced

1 head of broccoli, cut into florets

4 pak choi, tough base removed, then halved and leaves separated

50g podded edamame beans (about 100g in their pods)

Put the warm water, miso and soy into a bowl and combine to make a paste; set aside.

In a large lidded frying pan or wok, heat the coconut oil, add the garlic, ginger and chilli and cook for 1 minute before adding the cabbage and broccoli. Stir for a few minutes until they start to soften.

Stir in the miso paste then add a lid to the pan and cook for 2–3 minutes. Finally add the pak choi and edamame beans and cook for a further 2–3 minutes, or until all the veg are soft.

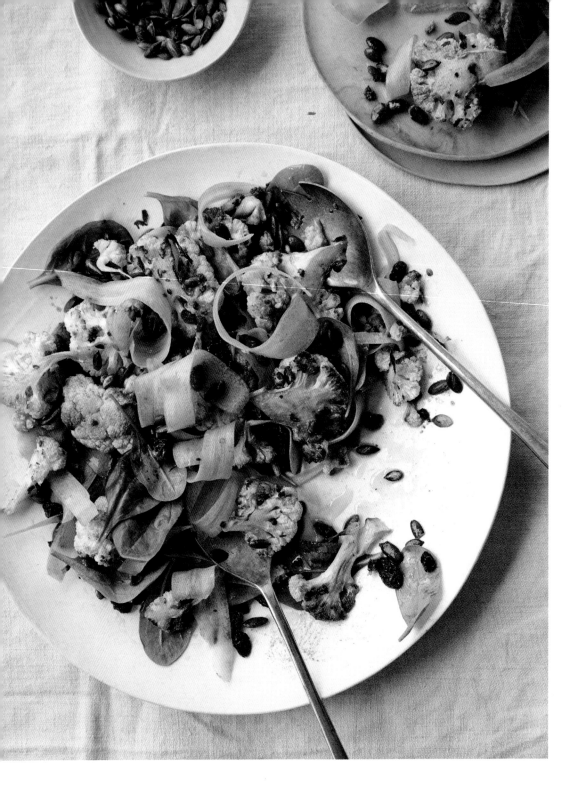

This is a great salad if you have time to put the oven on. I often add some quick pan-fried chicken or halloumi to turn this from a side salad into a main meal, but as a side dish it also goes beautifully with grilled salmon.

CRUNCHY CAULIFLOWER SALAD

SERVES 4

1 cauliflower, broken into 4–5cm florets

2 tbsp olive oil

1 tsp ground turmeric

1 tsp chilli flakes

½ tsp flaked salt

pinch of black pepper

100g spinach leaves

3 carrots, peeled into ribbons

1 tbsp raisins

2 tbsp Zingy Dressing (see page 239)

40g pumpkin seeds, toasted

Preheat the oven to 180°C fan/200°C/400°F/gas mark 6 and line a large baking tray with baking paper.

Put the cauliflower into a large bowl and toss with the olive oil, turmeric, chilli flakes and salt and pepper until all the florets are coated.

Spread the cauliflower out onto the lined baking tray and roast in the oven for 20 minutes, or until the florets are crispy and a knife easily glides through the thicker stems. You might like to stir them halfway through cooking to ensure they brown evenly.

When the cauliflower is ready, allow it to cool for a few minutes before transferring to a large bowl and tossing it with the spinach, carrots, raisins and dressing. Transfer to a serving dish or individual plates and scatter with the pumpkin seeds to finish.

Home-made pesto is a great healthy alternative to shop-bought pesto, which often contains added sugars and preservatives. I love this dish as it can be a protein source for vegetarians as well as a side dish. It will keep for 3 days in the fridge so don't be scared to double up and make a large batch. It makes a fab accompaniment to grilled lamb or tuna – or try serving it with a selection of other side dishes, antipasti-style.

PESTO BUTTER BEANS

SERVES 2

1 tbsp olive oil

1 x 400g tin butter beans, drained and rinsed

1–2 tbsp Sun-dried Tomato Pesto (see page 237)

grated zest and juice of 1 lemon

30g pumpkin seeds

salt and black pepper

Warm the olive oil in a large frying pan, add the butter beans and cook for 3 minutes, stirring frequently.

Add the pesto, lemon zest and juice and some black pepper. Taste and only add extra salt if necessary.

Meanwhile, toast the pumpkin seeds in a dry frying pan until lightly browned. Transfer the butter beans to a dish, sprinkle over the toasted seeds and serve.

This simple salad is a basic 'must have' to accompany almost any main meal. It's always nice to have some extra greens on the table; a portion of salad counts towards your five-a-day. You'll find a couple of dressing recipes in this chapter, both of which will liven up any salad.

You can combine any of the following ingredients to make your perfect salad but try to choose at least one item from each group.

SIMPLE GREEN SALAD

CHOOSE YOUR GREENS	CHOOSE YOUR HERBS	CHOOSE YOUR VEG	CHOOSE YOUR TOPPING
(2 large handfuls) Red or green lettuce, Cos lettuce, iceberg lettuce, rocket, baby spinach leaves, watercress	Mint, basil, parsley, thyme	2 spring onions, sliced ½ small red onion, sliced ½ cucumber, sliced 6 radishes, halved 10 cherry tomatoes, halved 1 carrot, grated ½ avocado, sliced	Dressing of choice Handful of croutons Feta cheese (25g per person) 1 tbsp toasted pine nuts 1 tbsp mixed nuts or seeds

Wash and dry the leaves – use a salad spinner if you have one, otherwise gently pat dry with some kitchen paper.

Toss the leaves, herbs and vegetables together with a little salad dressing. Transfer to a serving dish and finish with your chosen toppings.

Lentils are a good replacement for traditional carbs such as pasta or potatoes, or as a protein alternative for vegetarians; not to mention they keep in the cupboard for ages! I have thrown together a few of my favourite ingredients to make this a super-simple and tasty side salad, but it would also make an excellent lunch dish, with or without some crumbled feta cheese. You can cook the lentils yourself or buy ready-cooked lentils in pouches or tins to save time.

WARMING LENTIL AND SUN-DRIED TOMATO SALAD

SERVES 2

1 tbsp olive oil

1 small red onion, thinly sliced

160g puy lentils, rinsed

60g frozen peas

80g sun-dried tomatoes in olive oil, drained

1 tbsp balsamic vinegar

handful of mint leaves, chopped

small handful of crumbled feta (optional)

salt and black pepper

Tzatziki (see page 235), to serve

Heat the olive oil in a pan over a medium heat, add the sliced onion, with a pinch of salt to help them break down, and sauté for 5–7 minutes until softened.

Add the lentils to the pan and then cover them with boiling water. Bring to the boil, add a lid, then reduce to a low simmer and cook for 15–20 minutes until al dente. (If you are using pre-cooked lentils, simply add the lentils to the softened onions and continue with the following step.)

Remove the lid, add the frozen peas and cook for 2 minutes to allow them to thaw, then add the sun-dried tomatoes. If at this stage there is still excess water in the pan, drain it off then return to the heat.

Add the balsamic vinegar and season to taste with salt and pepper. Finally stir through the mint, reserving some to garnish. Scatter the feta cheese, if using, and remaining chopped mint over the top and serve with a dollop of Tzatziki.

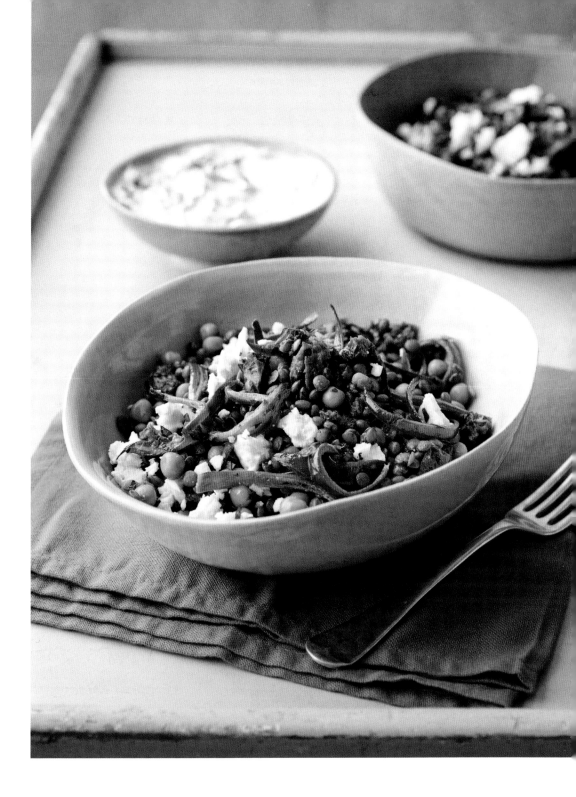

DIPS 4 WAYS

We all love a good dip but are you getting the most out of them? Dips aren't just for dipping so put down that giant bag of crisps! (Although they are great with my Flaxseed Crackers on page 212!)

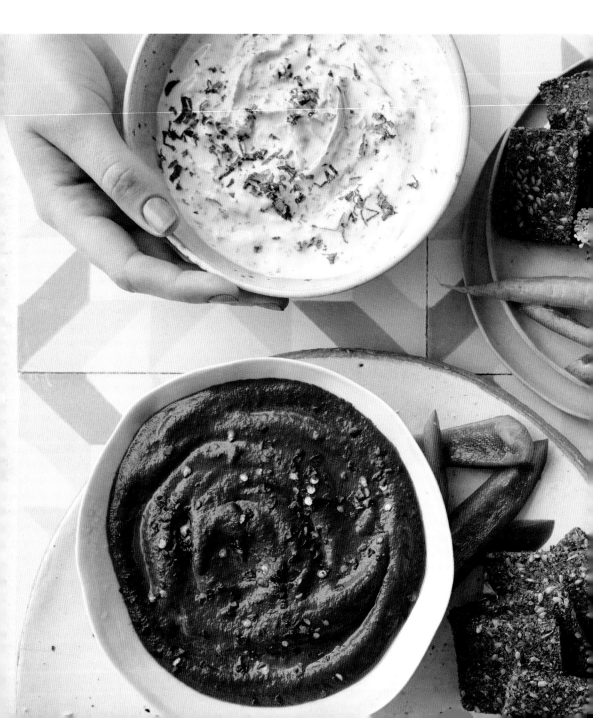

Jazz up your lunchbox – Add a dollop of dip to some cooked rice, pasta or quinoa and mix thoroughly to add a boost of flavour. Try this with the Beetroot Dip or Sun-dried Tomato Pesto.

Jazz up your porridge – People always forget that porridge can be savoury too! Get super-creative by stirring in your dip of choice; try a creamy tzatziki!

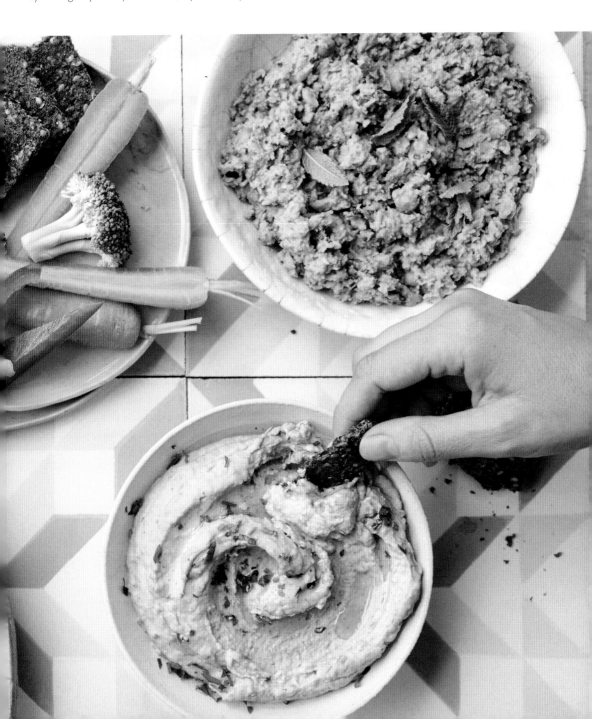

BEETROOT DIP

SERVES 4–6

300g cooked beetroot, roughly chopped

2 tbsp Greek yoghurt (or other plain yoghurt of choice)

2 tbsp lemon juice

1½ tbsp olive oil

1 garlic clove, very finely chopped

½ tsp chilli flakes, plus extra to garnish

½ tsp hot paprika

¼ tsp salt

black pepper

1–2 tbsp finely chopped coriander or parsley (optional)

The nutritional benefits of beetroot have been linked to various health benefits, from improved athletic stamina and blood flow to reduced blood pressure. Its bright purple colour tells you that it's good for you; the more colour the better! Try serving with my Quinoa Falafel (see page 161).

Put all the ingredients except the chopped herbs, if using, into a blender and blitz until smooth.

Taste and adjust the seasoning, adding more salt, pepper or lemon juice as needed. Transfer to a bowl and garnish with extra chilli flakes if you like, and the chopped herbs.

AUBERGINE HUMMUS

SERVES 4–6

2 aubergines, halved lengthways

5 tbsp olive oil, plus extra to serve

1 x 400g tin chickpeas, drained and rinsed

3 tbsp tahini

2 tbsp lemon juice

3 garlic cloves, very finely chopped

pinch of salt and black pepper

small handful of parsley, finely chopped

Two of my favourite things in life – aubergine and hummus – come together in this dip and I LOVE it! Just make sure the aubergine is cooked thoroughly. Serve with any main dish, with Flaxseed Crackers (see page 212) or with crunchy Parsnip and Avocado Chips (see page 222).

Preheat the oven to 200°C fan/220°C/425°F/gas mark 7. Put the aubergine halves cut side up on a baking tray. Drizzle over 1 tablespoon of olive oil. Bake in oven for 25 minutes, until browned and soft – a knife should pierce the flesh easily. Allow to cool.

When cool enough to handle, scoop out the aubergine flesh, discarding the skins. Blitz with the chickpeas, tahini, lemon juice, garlic, salt and pepper, until it all starts to break down, then gradually pour in the remaining 4 tablespoons of olive oil with the motor still running.

Taste and adjust the seasoning before transferring to a serving bowl. Scatter over the chopped parsley and drizzle with a little more oil.

TZATZIKI

SERVES 4

1 cucumber, peeled,
halved lengthways,
deseeded and grated

300g Greek yoghurt
(or use a vegan/lactose-
free option)

20g mint leaves,
finely chopped

2 garlic cloves, very
finely chopped

1 tbsp lemon juice,
or to taste

salt and black pepper

This Greek classic is great with crudités and Flaxseed Crackers (see page 212). It's also very good for jazzing up meat as well as vegetables. You can make it dairy-free by using coconut yoghurt, or use a fat-free Greek yoghurt to keep the fat content lower.

Put the grated cucumber in a sieve and set over a large bowl. Sprinkle ½ teaspoon of salt over it, mix through and then cover with a bowl or plate topped with a heavy weight (I use a tin). The excess water from the cucumber will drip out; this may take up to an hour.

When the cucumber is ready, add it to a bowl with the remaining ingredients. Stir to combine, then taste and adjust the seasoning with more salt, pepper or lemon juice, as needed.

PEA AND MINT PURÉE

SERVES 4

300g frozen peas

20g mint leaves, plus
a sprig to garnish

1 tbsp butter or olive oil

¼ tsp salt

good grinding of
black pepper

Peas are often underrated, but they are amazing in this dip. The colour screams vitality and the mint brings the taste to a whole new level. I often serve it with a salmon fillet – the colours and flavours work wonderfully. It's also a key side dish to the Fish (or Tofu) and Chips on page 168.

Place the peas in a pan of boiling water and cook for 3–4 minutes until tender. Drain the peas, reserving 2–3 tablespoons of their cooking water.

Blend the peas with the reserved cooking water, mint leaves, butter or oil and seasoning. Blitz to a smooth green purée. Taste and adjust the seasoning if necessary; you may want to add more mint to give it a bit more oomph. Transfer to a bowl and garnish with a mint sprig.

If you know someone who doesn't like sweet potato, introduce them to this purée first. It's beautiful and creamy and works well with family meals too as an addition to your vegetables. A few dollops of this on your plate will add a portion of carbohydrate to your main meal.

SWEET POTATO AND GARLIC PURÉE

SERVES 4

4 sweet potatoes (about 200g each), split in half

1 tbsp olive oil, plus extra for puréeing

1 head of garlic, top sliced off

½ tsp cayenne pepper

¼ tsp smoked paprika

salt and black pepper

Preheat the oven to 200°C fan/220°C/425°F/gas mark 7.

Take a large piece of foil or baking paper and place the sweet potatoes in the middle. Drizzle over the olive oil, add a pinch of salt, then fold up the foil to make a sealed packet. Place on a baking tray.

Bake for 1–1¼ hours, adding the garlic to the sweet potato parcel halfway through cooking. The potatoes and garlic will be ready when they have completely softened. Remove from the oven and set aside to cool.

When they are cool enough to handle, scoop the sweet potato flesh from the skins into a bowl, then add the garlic cloves squeezed from their skins, along with the cayenne pepper and paprika. Mash together until smooth – you may like to add another tablespoon of olive oil. Season to taste. (Alternatively, you can combine all the ingredients in a food processor for a really smooth purée.)

I love my sun-dried tomatoes; they're so rich in flavour that they really do jazz up any dish, adding a burst of vitamin C and lycopene, a powerful antioxidant. That's why I made this red pesto, which can be dairy-free for all to enjoy! I often mix this into rice, pasta and roasted vegetables, or drizzle over cooked chicken.

SUN-DRIED TOMATO PESTO

MAKES 1 SMALL JAR

50g pine nuts, toasted (or use cashews)

25g Parmesan (or use a lactose-free/vegan substitute), grated

60g basil leaves

30g sun-dried tomatoes in olive oil, drained

2 garlic cloves, very finely chopped

5 tbsp olive oil

2 tbsp lemon juice

salt and black pepper

Put the pine nuts into a food processor and blitz briefly before adding the Parmesan, basil, sun-dried tomatoes, garlic and half of the olive oil. Blitz until a coarse paste forms, then with the motor still running, slowly drizzle in the rest of the oil. Stir in the lemon juice and season to taste.

Transfer to a jar with a tight-fitting lid and store in the fridge until needed. With a layer of oil at the top of the jar, this will keep for up to 7 days.

Serve with my delicious sea bass recipe (see page 174). This dressing can also be used to jazz up a plain green salad or some steak and green beans. Or you could even enjoy it as a lovely dip for roasted new potatoes or parsnip fries. You can chop all the ingredients by hand and then mix together or, alternatively, give it all a quick blitz in the food processor.

SALSA VERDE

SERVES 6

50g mixed soft herbs, such as basil, parsley, mint, chives

1 garlic clove, very finely chopped

2 tbsp capers, drained and roughly chopped

2–3 anchovy fillets, thinly sliced

4 tbsp olive oil

2 tbsp red wine vinegar

1 tbsp Dijon mustard

salt and black pepper

If you are making this by hand pick the herbs from their stalks, then roughly chop in the centre of a large chopping board. Add the garlic, capers and anchovies on top and continue chopping and mixing it all together.

Scrape everything into a large bowl and stir in the olive oil, red wine vinegar and mustard. Taste and season with salt and pepper (you may not need salt if your anchovies are particularly salty). You can also add more oil or vinegar for a runnier salsa.

Alternatively, place everything a food processor and blitz until combined (leaving some texture). Taste and season as required. This will keep in the fridge in a jar with a tight-fitting lid for a few days.

TWO SALAD DRESSINGS

HERBY YOGHURT DRESSING

SERVES 2–3

125g Greek yoghurt (ideally full-fat)

¼ small red onion, finely diced (about 1 tbsp)

1 garlic clove, very finely chopped

juice of ½ lemon

dash of Worcestershire sauce (optional)

handful of parsley, roughly chopped

5–6 chives, roughly chopped

6 large sage leaves, roughly chopped

salt and black pepper

This works just as well with coconut yoghurt if you want to make a dairy-free version. I find this dressing also goes really well with roasted vegetables and chicken – it's not just for salads!

Put the yoghurt, onion, garlic, lemon juice, Worcestershire sauce, if using, and some seasoning into a food processor and blitz until smooth.

Add the fresh herbs and pulse slowly – you want to chop them up, but still keep some of their texture. Taste and adjust the seasoning.

Alternatively, you can combine all the ingredients by hand, taking care to chop the onion as finely as possible before adding to the yoghurt.

ZINGY DRESSING

SERVES 2

3 tbsp olive oil

juice of ½ lemon

1 garlic clove, very finely chopped

1 tsp Dijon mustard

1 tsp tamari or soy sauce

Dressings are a great way to add a boost of flavour to a whole range of dishes, not just salad leaves. This dressing is so simple and a classic must-have for any fresh salad.

Put all the ingredients into a small bowl and whisk together until they are emulsified (smoothly combined). Alternatively, put all the ingredients into a jar with a tight-fitting lid and shake vigorously.

Store in an airtight container in the fridge until needed – this dressing will keep for up to 3 days.

This is a super-rich spread and an excellent alternative to cheese for vegans. I love spreading this on my toast in the mornings!

CASHEW CHEESE SPREAD

MAKES 1 SMALL JAR

200g raw cashews, soaked for at least 2 hours (or overnight is fine), drained and rinsed

juice of 1 lemon

2 tbsp nutritional yeast

¼ tsp garlic powder (use more for a stronger garlic flavour or use 1 very finely chopped garlic clove instead)

½ tsp salt, or to taste

¼ tsp black pepper

180ml water

small handful of chives or basil (optional)

Put the cashews, lemon juice, nutritional yeast, garlic powder and salt and pepper into a food processor. Pulse until the cashews break down and they form a coarse, wet meal. Scrape the sides of the food processor down with a spatula from time to time.

With the motor running, drizzle in three-quarters of the water and blitz the cashews for about 10 seconds. Stop and scrape the machine down again.

Continue processing for a full 1–2 minutes, or until the cashew cheese is smooth and thick, adding a little extra water as needed. The consistency should be a little bit like hummus.

Taste and adjust the seasoning with salt, pepper or lemon juice. If you like, pulse in some fresh herbs, such as chives or basil.

Transfer to an airtight container and store in the fridge for up to 6 days. Cashew cheese also freezes well.

Go on, give it a go! If you are looking to reduce your sugar intake and you have ketchup every day, this is a good place to start.

TOMATO KETCHUP

MAKES 1 SMALL JAR

1 tsp olive oil

1 garlic clove, very finely chopped

200g tomato purée (not double concentrate)

2 tbsp apple cider vinegar or red wine vinegar

1 tsp dried oregano

1 tsp onion powder

salt and black pepper

Warm the olive oil in a small pan over a medium heat and sauté the garlic for 1 minute. Add all the remaining ingredients and stir together – if your paste is still quite thick add a few tablespoons of water. Turn up the heat and allow the sauce to bubble for a couple of minutes.

Transfer to a blender and blitz until smooth (or use a hand-held stick blender). Store in a glass jar in the fridge for 3–4 days.

Trust me: it is super-simple to make your own chocolate sauce. It also tastes better and you can adjust the sweetness to your liking by changing the percentage of chocolate you use. I recommend going for dark chocolate with at least 70% cocoa solids – you can always add a little honey or sweetener of choice for added sweetness if desired. Drizzle this sauce over berries and porridge – and dip nuts in it too.

CHOCOLATE SAUCE

SERVES 2

50g dark chocolate, broken into small pieces

2 tbsp milk of choice

1 tsp coconut flour (optional)

Put the chocolate and milk into a small pan and melt over a low heat.

When the chocolate has melted, stir until smooth. If you want a slightly thicker sauce, stir in the coconut flour to thicken the sauce further.

If you have the time, making your own nut butter is easy; you just need a good food processor. I love adding spices to mine for a natural sweetness – most nut butters on the shelves have added sugar and oil, so making your own is a fun way to ensure you know what is going in your food. This makes a delicious snack spread onto apple slices.

NUT BUTTER

MAKES 1 SMALL JAR

200g raw unsalted
almonds

1 tsp vanilla extract

1 tsp ground cinnamon

¼ tsp ground ginger

pinch of ground nutmeg

For a super-smooth butter you can remove the skins from the almonds: blanch them in hot water for 60 seconds and then drain, cool immediately in cold water and peel. Set aside to dry.

Preheat the oven to 180°C fan/200°C/400°F/gas mark 6 and line a baking tray with baking paper.

Spread the almonds on the tray and toast in the oven for 10 minutes. Let them cool for just a minute or so (they will be easier to blend when slightly warm).

Put the warm almonds into a food processor and blitz (unless you have a high-speed blender I would advise turning the blender off for a few seconds every minute or so to avoid the blender burning out). The almonds will take a while to turn into a butter. First they break up into crumbs, and then become creamy as their natural oils are released. Stop every now and then to scrape down the sides of the bowl (and to give the blender's motor a rest).

Eventually the almonds will resemble shop-bought almond butter. Now you can add in the rest of the ingredients before a final blitz to mix them in. Scrape into a clean jam jar and store in the fridge for up to 2 weeks.

This is an indulgent spread, but I say all good things in moderation!
If you make your own chocolate spread you can control the sugar and
pick a chocolate with a high cocoa solids percentage. Spreads on the
shop shelves often have extra ingredients in them to modify the texture
and increase their shelf life, so home-made is always a better option.
I love to smother this spread onto a seeded cracker!

CHOCOLATE SPREAD

MAKES 500ML

40g hazelnuts

60g honey or maple syrup

450g dark chocolate
(at least 70–85% cocoa
solids), broken into small
pieces

225ml double cream

100g unsalted butter,
cubed

pinch of salt

Preheat the oven to 180°C fan/200°C/400°F/gas mark 6.

Spread the hazelnuts onto a baking tray and toast in the oven for
10 minutes, or until golden. Leave to cool for a few minutes, then tip
onto a clean tea towel and rub them until their skins fall off.

Place the skinned nuts and honey or maple syrup in a food processor
and blitz until a paste forms.

Meanwhile, set up a bain marie to melt your chocolate: place a
heatproof bowl over a small pan of simmering water, making sure
the base of the bowl doesn't touch the water. Put the chocolate into
the bowl and leave it to melt into a pool of liquid.

Add the cream and butter to the chocolate, give it a good stir and
allow it to melt completely. Take the bowl off the heat and fold in the
hazelnut-honey paste and a pinch of salt.

Pour into a clean jar or jars, cool and then transfer to the fridge,
where it will keep for a couple of weeks. This is best served at room
temperature (to make spreading easier) so remove from the fridge
5–10 minutes before serving.

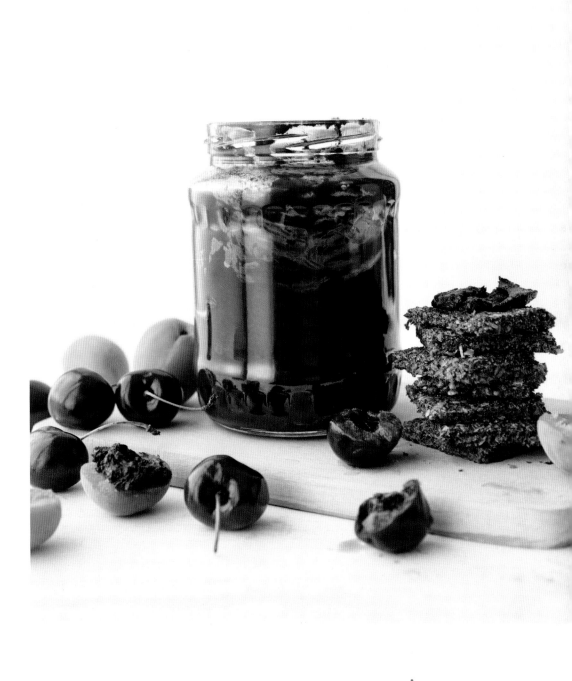

REFERENCES

MY PHILOSOPHY

1. www.mintel.com/press-centre/food-and-drink/brits-lose-count-of-their-calories-over-a-third-of-brits-dont-know-how-many-calories-they-consume-on-a-typical-day
2. Sainsbury. (2017). Eat Well Well Move Well Live Well Report. Available: www.j-sainsbury.co.uk/~/media/Files/S/Sainsburys/documents/making-a-difference/sainsburys-eat-well-move-well-live-well-report.pdf. Last accessed 26th June 2017.

NOURISHMENT

1. www.ncbi.nlm.nih.gov/pmc/articles/PMC524030
2. www.nutrition.org.uk/nutritionscience/nutrients-food-and-ingredients/protein.html
3. www.ncbi.nlm.nih.gov/pubmed/15466943
4. www.ncbi.nlm.nih.gov/pubmed/25169440
5. www.ncbi.nlm.nih.gov/pmc/articles/PMC4180248
6. www.ncbi.nlm.nih.gov/pubmed/20711407
7. www.jama.jamanetwork.com/journals/jama/fullarticle/201882
8. www.malnutritiontaskforce.org.uk/resources/malnutrition-factsheet
9. www.cochrane.org/CD011737/VASC_effect-of-cutting-down-on-the-saturated-fat-we-eat-on-our-risk-of-heart-disease
10. www.ncbi.nlm.nih.gov/pubmed/27457635
11. www.ncbi.nlm.nih.gov/pubmed/24860193
12. www.sciencedirect.com/science/article/pii/S0753332206002435
13. www.ncbi.nlm.nih.gov/pubmed/19022225
14. www.ncbi.nlm.nih.gov/pubmed/22216328
15. www.ncbi.nlm.nih.gov/pubmed/10448517
16. www.ncbi.nlm.nih.gov/pubmed/27412317
17. www.ncbi.nlm.nih.gov/pubmed/23642776
    www.ncbi.nlm.nih.gov/pubmed/23510814
    www.ncbi.nlm.nih.gov/pubmed/26061039
18. www.ncbi.nlm.nih.gov/pubmed/24285687
    www.ncbi.nlm.nih.gov/pubmed/19640950
19. www.ncbi.nlm.nih.gov/pubmed/24528693

20. www.ncbi.nlm.nih.gov/pubmed/24246205
21. www.ncbi.nlm.nih.gov/pubmed/21631511
22. www.ncbi.nlm.nih.gov/pubmed/20458092
23. www.ncbi.nlm.nih.gov/pubmed/24710915
24. www.lnds.nhs.uk/Library/DietaryadviceforincreasingfibreOct15.pdf
25. Enders, G (2014). GUT. London: Scribe. 169–170
26. https//epi.grants.cancer.gov/diet/usualintakes/pop/2001–04/added_sugars.html
27. www.apa.org/monitor/2013/10/hunger.aspx
28. www.ncbi.nlm.nih.gov/pmc/articles/PMC4241367
29. www.ncbi.nlm.nih.gov/pmc/articles/PMC1402378
30. www.ncbi.nlm.nih.gov/pubmed/24447775
31. www.ncbi.nlm.nih.gov/pubmed/18834505
    www.ncbi.nlm.nih.gov/pubmed/9252488
    www.ncbi.nlm.nih.gov/pubmed/20048505
    www.ncbi.nlm.nih.gov/pubmed/10198297
32. www.ncbi.nlm.nih.gov/pubmed/18834505

FOOD CLINIC

1. https//link.springer.com/article/10.1007/s40519-017-0364-2
2. www.orthorexia.com
3. www.health.harvard.edu/staying-healthy/mindful-eating
4. www.mdpi.com/2072-6643/8/8/479/htm
5. www.ncbi.nlm.nih.gov/pubmed/10408315

RE-NOURISH MENU

1. www.ncbi.nlm.nih.gov/pubmed/19930003
   www.ncbi.nlm.nih.gov/pubmed/17381386
   www.ncbi.nlm.nih.gov/pubmed/16634838
2. www.ncbi.nlm.nih.gov/pmc/articles/PMC3995184
3. www.ncbi.nlm.nih.gov/pmc/articles/PMC3633300
4. www.ncbi.nlm.nih.gov/pubmed/22481014
5. www.nhs.uk/Livewell/Goodfood/Pages/food-labelling.aspx
6. www.soilassociation.org/certification/market-research-and-data/the-organic-market-report

INDEX

ACKNOWLEDGEMENTS

I am so incredibly grateful to be able to share my passion for nutrition with you all in the form of this, my very own book. I honestly never dreamed that I would have the opportunity to reach so many people who want to see nutrition integral to living a fulfilled life. There are so many people who have supported me in my own journey, culminating in the writing of this book and, although writing a few words will never really repay their faith in me, I hope it goes some way to telling them how truly grateful I am.

The first step I took in studying nutrition was at The University of Roehampton where, if it weren't for my lecturers, especially Dr Sue Reeves RNutr, Yvonne Wake RNutr and Dr Patrick Brady enduring the many hours of my never-ending desire to learn, my career may not have progressed the way it has. I hope they will continue to be a constant source of knowledge and guidance and I am forever grateful for their priceless time invested me.

Thank you to everyone at Yellow Kite and Hodder for believing in me. It has been an honour to work with such a dedicated publisher who shares my real passion for health. However, I must say a special thank you to Lauren who first approached me and whose unwavering positive support has always made me feel there was no better home for *Re-Nourish*.

The collaborative and creative process in bringing everything together in this book has taken the imagination of so many people. The extraordinary contribution of Laura and Lauren for making the process so wonderfully uncomplicated and refining my work deserves an enormous thank you.

Thank you also Tamin, Sarah, Ruth and Stephanie for capturing me and my recipes so beautifully, Rosie, Jess, Esther and Olivia for their meticulous styling, hair and makeup artists Ingrid and Ami, Becca and Caitriona for their PR and marketing prowess and Abi for designing this gorgeous book.

Thank you to kitchen extraordinaire Ceri, who assisted me in experimenting and critically appraising my recipes for months.

Over the years, I am so lucky to have built a support network of so many nutrition and health professionals. However, I tasked Registered Dietitian Jen Low to double-check my work and without her wise words and distinct contribution, this book would not have been as far-reaching as it is.

Thank you Cath and Vanessa at Curtis Brown whose experience and profound professionalism is invaluable.

I have also been fortunate to find a great number of determined people to assist me in everything I do. A particular thank you to Bethany for being my right-hand woman throughout this process and Daisy for her valuable contribution.

The reason I embarked on a career in nutrition was an interest in just how important a role nutrition plays in life. I am proud to have built a special community of clients, and with the rise in social media, I am now lucky enough to be able share my passion and philosophy with people all over the world. The endless kindness and support you show me every day only motivates me to believe in it more and share the basic nutrition knowledge everyone deserves.

Thank you to my best friend Tanya who has stood by me every turn of my unpredictable life in London and to my family and friends Alice, Steph, Laura, Nicky, Flora, Tessa, Becki and Chessie for being there and understanding the ups and downs.

From the bottom my heart, thank you to my partner Billy. I will be forever grateful for us finding one another with no words coming close to sharing how lucky I am to have his unrelenting love for everything I do.

Last but by no means least, I would like to thank my Grandma Jean who is watching over my every move. She will always be my biggest inspiration and I hope to have made her proud.

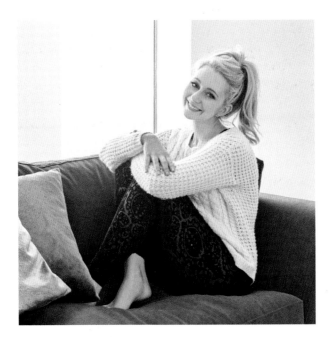

First published in Great Britain in 2017 by Yellow Kite
An imprint of Hodder & Stoughton
An Hachette UK company

1

The advice herein is not intended to replace the services of trained health and fitness
professionals, or be a substitute for medical advice. You are advised to consult with
your healthcare professional with regards to matters relating to your health, and in
particular regarding matters that may require diagnosis or medical attention.

A CIP catalogue record for this title is available from the British Library

Trade Paperback ISBN 978 1 473 66176 9
eBook ISBN 978 1 473 66177 6

Editor: Lauren Whelan
Project Editor: Laura Herring
Design and art direction: HART STUDIO
Photography: Tamin Jones
Prop styling: Olivia Wardle
Food styling: Rosie Reynolds
Shoot Producer: Ruth Ferrier
Peer Review: Jennifer Low
Recipe Testing: Ceri Jones

Colour origination by Born
Printed in China by 1010 Printing Co Ltd

Hodder & Stoughton policy is to use papers that are natural, renewable and
recyclable products and made from wood grown in sustainable forests. The logging
and manufacturing processes are expected to conform to the environmental
regulations of the country of origin.

Yellow Kite
Hodder & Stoughton Ltd
Carmelite House
50 Victoria Embankment
London
EC4Y 0DZ

www.yellowkitebooks.co.uk
www.hodder.co.uk